THE HEALING ENERGIES OF EARTH

LIZ SIMPSON

THE HEALING ENERGIES OF EARTH

JOURNEY EDITIONS

Boston - Tokyo - Singapore

First published in the United States in 2000 by Journey Editions, an imprint of Periplus Editions (HK) Ltd., with editorial offices at 153 Milk Street, Boston, Massachusetts 02109.

Library of Congress Card Number: 99-068814

ISBN: 1-58290-013-2

Distributed by

USA
Tuttle Publishing
Distribution Center
Airport Industrial Park
364 Innovation Drive
North Clarendon, VT 05759-9436
Tel: (802) 773-8930
Tel: (800) 526-2778

Canada
Raincoast Books
8680 Cambie Street
Vancouver, British Columbia
V6P 6M9
Tel: (604) 323-7100
Fax: (604) 323-2600

Japan
Tuttle Shuppan
RK Building, 2nd Floor
2-13-10 Shimo-Meguro, Meguro-Ku
Tokyo 153 0064
Tel: (03) 5437-0171
Fax: (03) 5437-0755

Southeast Asia (excluding Singapore and Malaysia)
Berkeley Books Pte Ltd
5 Little Road #08-01
Singapore 536983
Tel: (65) 280-1330
Fax: (65) 280-6290

First edition
06 05 04 03 02 01 00   10 9 8 7 6 5 4 3 2 1

Design by Matt Moate

Printed in Italy

To Ann
For the healing energy you bring to our friendship

Caution
The techniques, ideas, and suggestions in this book are to be used at the reader's sole discretion and risk. Always observe the cautions given, and consult a doctor if you are in doubt about a medical condition.

A Note from the Author

While Earth is a separate entity to us, our bodies are comprised of and depend on the same chemical compounds that form it: we are part of Earth just as it is part of us. This connection is explained archetypally through the universal concept of Earth as the Great Mother goddess, Gaia, stemming from our ancestors' understanding of the interdependent relationship between this planet and its inhabitants. Earlier civilizations revered the Earth and the natural processes that ensured the continued existence of humankind. Unfortunately, this was not to last as Earth-focused spiritual practices were engulfed by patriarchal religions. In many cultures, wise women were demonized for showing innate sensitivity to Nature and its healing gifts. At the height of this persecution sprang the obsession with exploiting Earth's resources for economic gain: modern science became Master of the Universe. It is therefore no surprise that greater interest in esoteric practices and concern for the environment have developed simultaneously with the re-introduction of women into positions of power. Ironically, it is through revolutionary discoveries in physics that the Newtonian concept of a material and mechanical Universe is being turned on its head: the "new" physics offers us an insight into phenomena previously considered magical, and therefore "unscientific".

This book allows you to tap in to many beliefs and practices through which our ancestors demonstrated respect for the Earth, as well as outlining the scientific basis behind our shared resonance. It also explores controversial theories, such as how the Earth and her inhabitants constitute the holographic nature of a living Universe: that which some call "God". I hope that, with a greater understanding of Earth and our relationship to it, you will be able to prolong both your own life and that of Gaia and improve your health — be it mental, physical, or spiritual — and that of our beautiful but fragile planet.

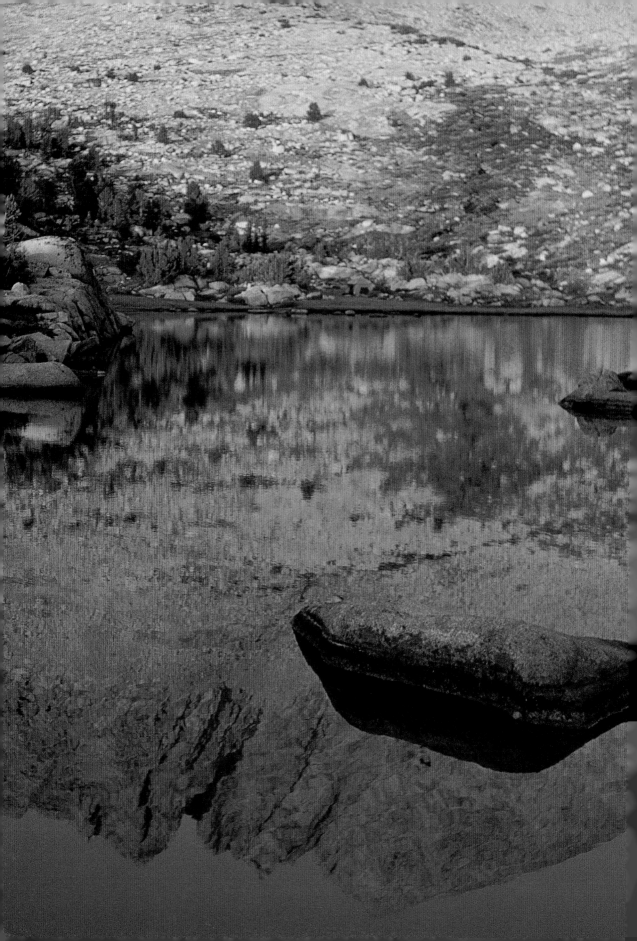

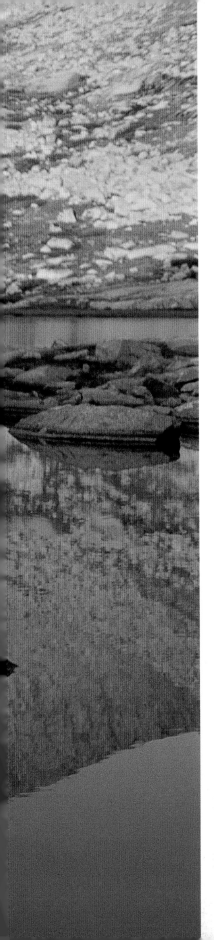

Contents

Introduction

Imagine that you have been transported back — not just physically but intellectually — to the world of our early forebears, when daily life was dictated by the seasons and the natural cycle of each day, when the night skies were lit by only the Moon and the stars and were free from the orange glow of the cities. Picture a life of relative silence, where the only ambient noises were the sounds of Nature: birdsong; the rustling of small animals; or the buzzing of bees.

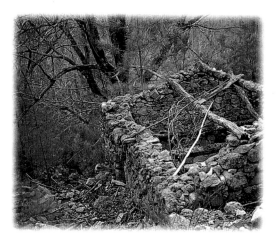

René Descartes is commonly regarded as the founder of modern philosophy. He argued that anything that could not be proven must be doubted. He proposed a mechanistic basis for his theory of dualism, where mind and matter were separate and, as such, worked independently of the other. He also shared the view of Sir Francis Bacon that the aim of science was to "render ourselves the masters and possessors of nature".

Imagine that your education has been free from the rational influence of Descartes, French philosopher (1596-1650), whose writings on mind and matter have encouraged the dichotomy of our intellects and physical selves (see left). Instead, all your energies are devoted to survival. Bread cannot be bought from a supermarket: you have to grow the wheat that depends on nourishment from the soil and the interventions of the Sun and rain. In your need to understand and predict what appears to be inexplicable and uncontrollable — the aim of modern science — you invest these processes with personalities in the guise of gods, goddesses, and Earth spirits, all of which must be appeased.

It is from such a world that a connected, interdependent, animistic, and more intuitive understanding of our relationship with the Earth has developed. It is this understanding that many are now trying to rediscover by acknowledging the importance of the spiritual alongside the material. Unfortunately there are many more physical and intellectual barriers impinging on this understanding than there were, particularly concerning the noise and frenetic pace of modern, Western life, which interferes with our innate ability to tap in to our supersensory awareness. In her book, *Where Science and Magic Meet*, psychologist Serena Roney-Dougal considers evidence suggesting that the subconscious mind processes and retains every item of information we are exposed to, not just in terms of our five senses but also in terms of our wider perception, commonly known as our sixth sense. She reveals that some researchers believe the reason behind our dreaming is to enable the brain to offload this extraneous information in the same way that a computer dumps unwanted programs. However, for many of us our dreams are the only connection we have with the symbolic language of the subconscious. While many people resist the notion of a sixth sense, experiences suggest otherwise, with urges to act on hunches, occasions of déjà vu, or the sense of being watched.

While the science of attention is relatively new in the field of cognitive psychology, it has become clear that our brains have a filtering system to avoid sensory saturation. Nonetheless, this system has been found to be more complex and related to a greater variety of levels and nervous system processes than was first thought.

In terms of modern science, early civilizations drew on a fanciful set of explanations to account for phenomena they could not explain. Nonetheless, this does not render the phenomena themselves any less real or detectable in those rare, silent moments when we push the modern world aside and commune with Nature. What was once thought magical and mysterious may simply be explained as knowledge that comes from the subconscious mind. Our earliest ancestors seem to have had access to certain understandings that, with today's sophisticated technical equipment, we have only been able to replicate or verify relatively recently. This was undoubtedly because their societies allowed them to foster an awareness of the natural (see right) way of things — their intuitive knowledge or Universal Laws — instead of drowning it in the cacophony of noise and plethora of tasks that fill our lives today.

Self-development guru, Wayne Dyer, states: "When you believe it, you'll see it." In scientific parlance this is often called the Experimenter Effect, meaning that when a researcher anticipates a certain result within an experiment, it is this result they achieve. This phenomenon has never been more profoundly demonstrated than in the physics laboratories of quantum scientists,

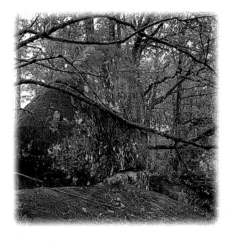

The word "natural" used throughout this book implies neither that it is "good" nor "bad". Many things that are "natural" — like snake venom and certain toxic plants — can be deadly to humans. This word is merely used to describe a process or phenomenon that relates to, or has been produced by, Nature rather than humans.

who have discovered that all matter is predisposed to exist in the simultaneous states of particles (concrete, localized, and physical) and waves (invisible, non-local, and energetic). This was the concept behind Einstein's declaration that matter and energy are two sides of the same coin. Whichever form atomic material takes depends on how the researcher chooses to measure it, that is, if the viewer anticipates measuring an electron as a particle they will see a particle, but if they expect to measure it as a wave, they will experience a wave. This could well be scientific validity for the age-old spiritual axiom that we create our own reality with our thoughts, completely overturning the Cartesian notion of an orderly and predictable cause-and-effect world. The paradox of both "being" (particle state) and "becoming" (wave state) also helps to explain various so-called magical phenomena, such as divination and precognition.

Up until the eighteenth century, when education was predominately in the hands of the Church, physics and the energetics of science were used to explain and promote Christianity. The Enlightenment brought with it the increasing secularization of knowledge, with scientists breaking away from the influence of the Church to focus on the directly tangible, physical aspects of the Universe. They steered clear of the more energetic aspects to avoid offending the Church and in an effort to base their knowledge on fact not faith. Both of these approaches to science resulted in the suppression of many ancient traditions and beliefs that embraced an energetic appreciation of our environment and life itself. It has taken until the first quarter of the twentieth century for new science to establish that the Universe has a dual nature of both matter and energy.

Today people talk of a "paradigm shift" taking place. Interestingly, the word paradigm, relating to the thoughts, perceptions, and values that comprise our version of what we call reality, comes from the Greek *paradeiknynai* — *para* meaning beyond and *deiknynai* meaning to show, i.e. beyond the material. The 300-

year-old Cartesian and Newtonian conditioning that has influenced our perceptions so profoundly appears to be undergoing a paradigm shift, our world — or Universe — being characterized as a system of patterns that are organic, indivisible, and ecological. This is the very same intuitive wisdom our ancestors embraced millennia ago in their awareness of a living environment and humankind's interdependent relationship with it.

But where did the supreme knowledge of our ancestors originate from? What wellspring of understanding did they tap in to when listening to their subconscious? From where does what Jung termed the Collective Unconscious originate? It is here that the theory of one very important universal pattern — the interconnectedness between God, ourselves, and our earthly home becomes relevant. It amalgamates spiritual and philosophical beliefs as well as new science, concentrating on what we now understand to be the nature of the brain and memory. This hypothesis underpins much of this book, which you may accept, amend, or reject.

In the *Timaeus*, the Greek philosopher Plato (c.428-348BC) described explicitly how everything that exists is ultimately a single being, an omnipresent Higher Power, call it God, the Universal Mind, Universal Life Force, Great Spirit, or Cosmic Consciousness. Plato's work also discusses the idea of the soul as the synthesis of and intermediary between the eternally unchanging Essence of the Universe (what quantum physicists might refer to as wave state) and the divisible, changing Existence of the physical world (particle state). Let us take this notion a stage further and consider the Universe to be the mind of God, with whom we are bound together in a single, holographic reality in the same way that many scientists now believe memories are held in the human brain. In the nineteenth century, French physiologist, Pierre Flourens, presented his theory that the brain acted as an entity and not as the interaction of separate parts. British physicist David Bohm, and other theorists, now accept Flourens' hypothesis, given experiments that demonstrate that — like a hologram — every part

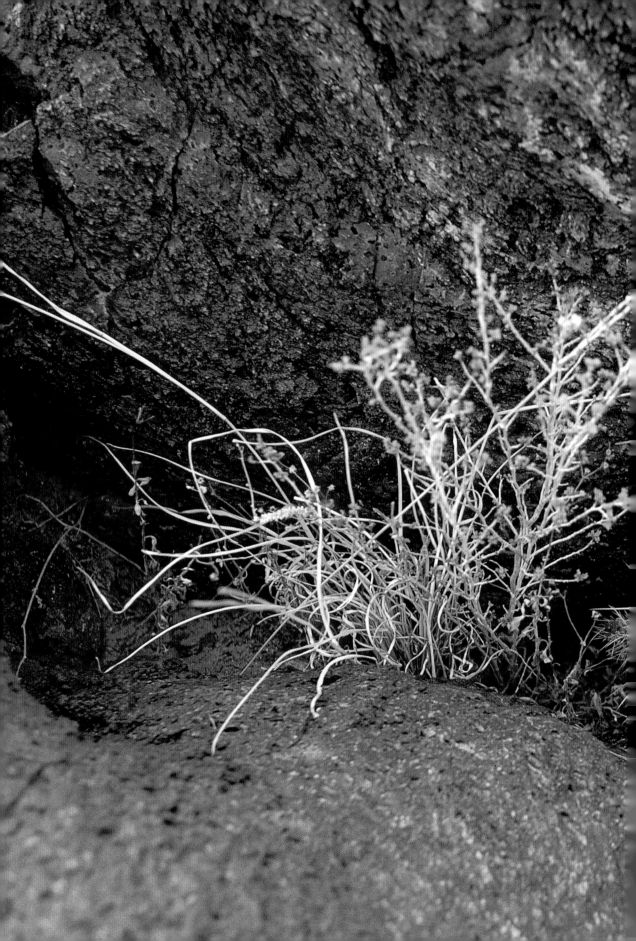

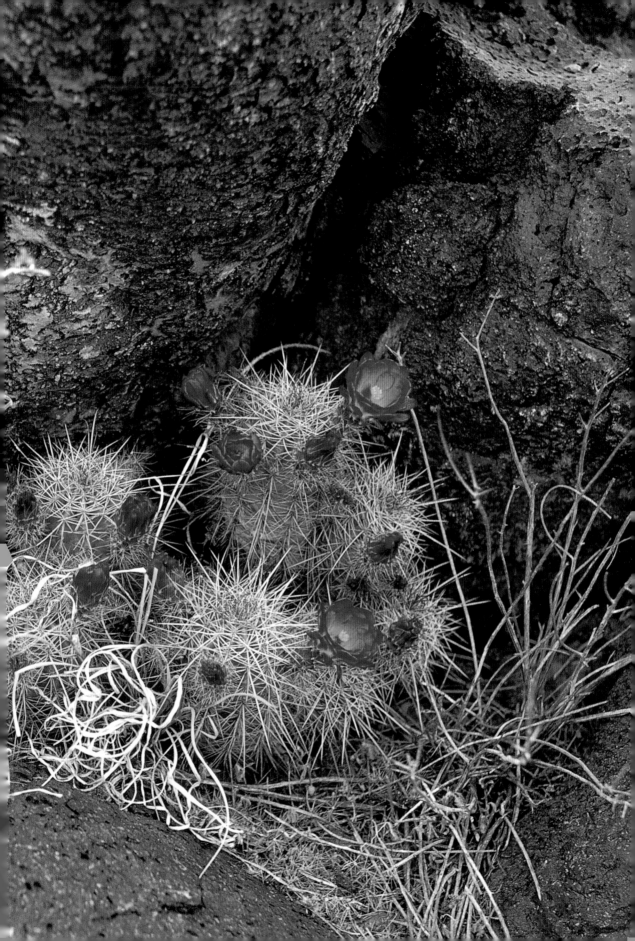

of the brain appears to include all memories. A hologram is a photograph that is produced when two parts of a split laser beam interfere with one another. The ensuing pattern is recorded on a photographic plate, resulting in a three-dimensional image when illuminated in a particular way. An amazing property of a holographic image is that if you break it each one of the resulting parts retains the same, albeit less detailed, picture as the original whole.

What if the Universe were indeed the mind of God, operating as a holographic entity so that each part of the macrocosm is a perfect, though perhaps less distinct, mirror image of the whole? This would mean that we are all of the same matter — and hence share the same characteristics — as the planets, the stars, this Earth, the rivers and oceans, and each blade of grass or species of bird. Within this holographic model, as is the case with scientifically produced holograms, the further the division is made from the original, the less detail is retained: human beings could represent the first, near perfect, level of holographic cloning; animals and birds could be a level further down or away from God, followed by insects, bacteria, rocks, water, and so on. As with the hologram, no part of the original (i.e. God or the Universal Mind) is lost, it is just a little less refined. This would mean that God, humankind, indeed everything in existence, animate or inanimate, is harmoniously interconnected. There is no separation, no need to "find" God or come back to Him/Her in death because God lives in us all. This would account for why psychologists — through a rather obscure psychological theory called Signal Detection Theory (SDT) — as well as philosophers down the centuries, have stated that, theoretically at least, our every thought or action can affect every other thing in the Universe. We have the potential to know everything that ever has been, is, or will be; we have the ability to know the mind of God.

Perhaps our earliest ancestors operated on this basis, in harmony with their world and everything in it. It is this that we are seeking to rediscover. This theory therefore supports the suggestion made by countless environmentalists that in polluting and destroying Earth we are contaminating and destroying ourselves and a part of God. Our relationship with Earth is becoming increasingly parasitic: we rip out and burn her fossil fuels; decimate her forests and pollute her rivers and oceans; murder animals for sport or vanity; we divest the soil of every ounce of goodness and poison it with chemicals. Only seldom do we take the time to gaze in awe and appreciation at the way Mother Earth continues to create new life from death and destruction.

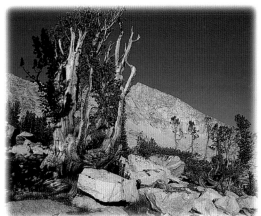

In this book I steer a middle course between the reductionist view of the orthodox sciences and the romantic but often impractical thinking of some New Age advocates. *The Healing Energies of Earth* integrates ancient and modern ways of looking at Gaia, the Mother Goddess, and discusses each based on a holistic understanding of Earth's energies. However, it is also a practical book, which suggests how you might improve your personal health and wellbeing, offering guidance on physical, emotional, and spiritual self-healing. It demonstrates how our existence on this planet can be enhanced on an individual and global scale for, as our only home, we have a responsibility to care for her if we want to continue to benefit from her healing powers and energies.

Chapter One, *Earth Science*, considers the cosmology, geology, geography, and physics of this planet, discussing both the physical nature, or matter, of Earth and her intangible, electromagnetic nature. It demonstrates that the two are merely flipsides of the same reality. Both concepts support the interrelationship between humankind and this planet where we are born, where we live, and die. Perhaps it is no coincidence that biologist James Lovelock hypothesized that Earth is a self-regulating, living organism only a few years after humankind first saw the awe-inspiring pictures of this planet seen from space by the 1968 US Apollo 8 mission. Our beautiful globe, suspended against a backdrop of inky black, like a Christmas tree bauble, revealed itself to be far more fragile and vulnerable than humankind had believed. How ironic that the greatest threat to her continuing existence should come not from external influences but from the human race: we should not abuse Earth's magnificent propensity to maintain homeostasis, or equilibrium.

Chapter Two, *Sacred Earth*, considers our planet from a historical and mythological perspective. It examines a number of creation myths and the concept of the Earth as the archetypal Good Mother, as well as the ancient rituals, practices, and belief systems now finding support within some of the newer scientific disciplines. It discusses the global extent of animism and shamanism and how the Roman Catholic Church, from the Middle Ages to the Age of Reason in the eighteenth century and beyond, has denied the existence of psychic abilities or beliefs, crushing pagan practices such as Wicca or the Old Religion while building its churches on their sacred sites and adopting their festivals. The Earth has been our creative canvas since the dawn of history, with examples still evident through the mysterious Nazca lines in Peru, the Lascaux cave paintings in France, or ground sculptures in the USA and Australia. Early civilizations fashioned temples and burial sites from specific materials. Despite their lack of technical equipment did ancient peoples know a great deal more about the acoustical properties of various minerals than was previously believed? This chapter looks at some examples. Developing the concept of "as above, so below", we also compare the human subtle energy system — meridians and chakras — with what we know about Earth energies, in the form, for example, of ley lines and the Earth's sacred places.

Chapter Three, *Ancient Practices*, takes an anthropological approach and offers an overview of how the art and science of human activities such as geomancy, dowsing, and making spiritual journeys of self-discovery, have developed from early people's intuitive understanding of our relationship with Earth. In Chapter Four, *You and Your Earth,* the most practical of these ancient practices are examined in detail, demonstrating how you can successfully and usefully integrate them into your daily life, in order to live more harmoniously within your environment. Finally, Chapter Five, *This Healing Earth,* focuses on various ways to heal and beautify yourself using different aspects of Earth's energies, from crystals for physical, emotional, and spiritual healing to the magic of minerals for deep cleansing and detoxifying. The book concludes with step-by-step instructions on how to create your own sacred space.

If, as quantum physics and ancient spiritual beliefs suggest, we create our own reality through the power of our minds, then it has never been more important to turn our attention to what we as individuals can do to ensure a healthy future for this planet. The holographic model of the Universe, I believe, can give us the incentive to achieve this: through it we know that each one of us is an integral part of the whole; what we think, do, or fail to do, has a very real impact on the existence of Earth. If we truly desire in our hearts, as well as our minds, to leave her — and ourselves — as vibrant and as beautiful as she was at our births, to replace domination and destruction with harmony and respect, then that intention will create a future reality of which we can all be proud. That purpose starts here and now, with ourselves.

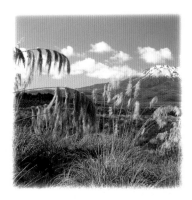

Earth Science

Star Trek's Captain Kirk may have considered space to be the final frontier, but there remains much mystery far closer to home, beneath our feet, in the very rocks and soil. It extends to meet the heavens as mountains and it holds in its belly a subterranean world.

In today's "global village" there may seem little left to explore. Geographically this may be true, but perhaps the most profound discovery involves rekindling our relationship with the Earth goddess Gaia, to rediscover the energetic relationship that sustained our ancestors physically, psychologically, and spiritually. Ancient peoples revered the sacredness of this Earth. They acknowledged the reciprocal relationship and responsibility, the interdependence between all life and our earthly home, intuitively understanding that good health is inextricably bound up with environment. Not until James Lovelock postulated the Gaia Hypothesis was the idea of Earth as a living entity taken seriously (see pp.48-9).

This chapter begins by looking at the matter of planet Earth in terms of what is tangible: the dynamic nature of geology and geography; the history contained in rock formations; the natural power that humankind harnesses but remains powerless to control. It then explores the subtler electromagnetic properties and resonance of Earth and outlines some of their health implications.

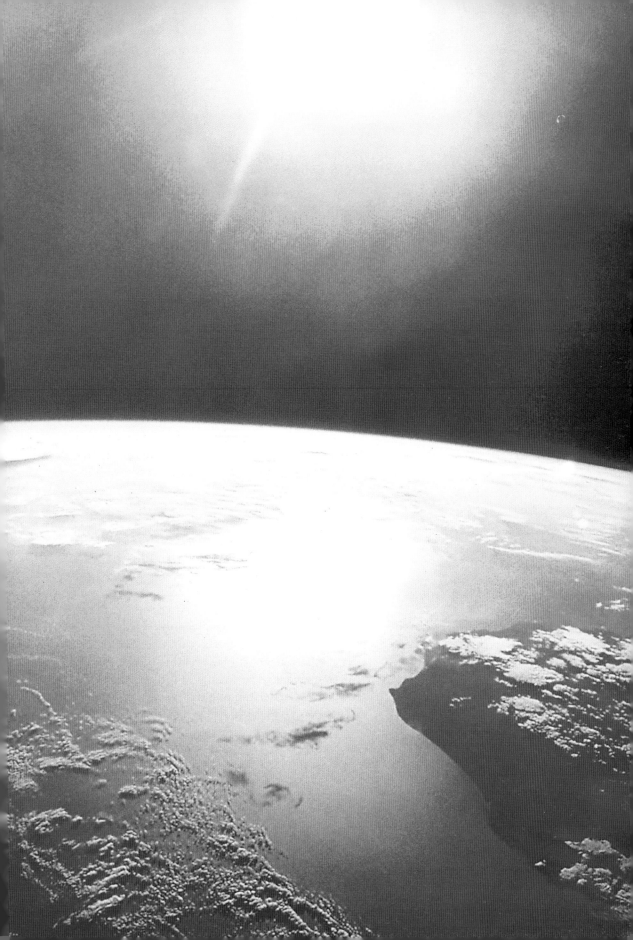

The Origins of the Universe

The Big Bang Theory, about the origins of the known Universe, harmonizes the concepts of both energy and matter. In some ways it is the scientific equivalent of numerous creation myths (see pp.44-9), which wove stories around the belief that what we now conceive as the Universe was once an empty void. Some time between 10 and 20 billion years ago conditions, still largely shrouded in mystery, produced a thermonuclear explosion fusing subatomic particles into the chemical elements, simultaneously creating matter, gravity, elec-

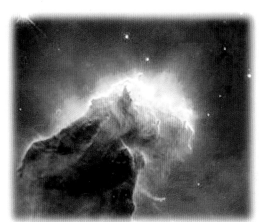

tromagnetism, and time. The first of these elements were hydrogen and helium, which, as they expanded and cooled over millions of years, condensed into the stars and galaxies.

Cosmologists currently consider the Universe to consist of matter, ranging from the visible — ordinary atomic matter forming stars, dust, and gas — to the much greater expanse of invisible dark matter, or the energy of space, whose identity is still unclear. So-called empty space is actually filled with "virtual" particles that pop in and out of existence too quickly to be detected directly. Contrary to established belief, cosmologists are finding that this form of energy is expanding, demonstrating a notion that even Einstein distrusted ("The biggest mistake of my life"): that the Universe is dynamic. It may even prove to be bigger and emptier than anyone originally thought.

A Star is Born

Although the oldest rocks on this planet are thought to date from 3.7 billion years ago, current theories postulate that the formation of our solar system took place about 4.6 billion years ago, when a vast cloud of interstellar dust and gases began to compress gravitationally until it formed a dense rotating mass, which expanded, producing the Sun and the planets. During its period of formation, the Earth's composition separated into an outermost thin crust on a pliant mantle and a core of iron and nickel that has an outer fluid zone around a solid centre. In some areas of the ocean floor the crust is only 5 km (3 miles) thick, whereas under the continents it is between 35 and 50 km (21 and 31 miles) thick. The mantle is approximately 2,800 km (1,740 miles) thick and the core of the Earth almost 7,000 km (4,350 miles) in diameter — representing one-third of the total mass, but only one-sixth of the volume. Most of the three layers of Earth are made up of rock-forming minerals. In a few cases these comprise a single mineral, such as pure marble, but in the majority of cases they are an amalgamation of two or more. The Earth is not completely spherical but bulges, the diameter at the equator being slightly longer than at the poles.

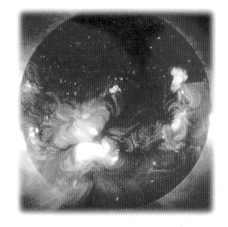

The Earth is one of nine planets orbiting the Sun in our solar system. While life in a form we cannot comprehend may exist on another planet, the view of Earth from space illustrates its unique, beauteous existence. Unlike its closest neighbours, Mars and Venus, the Earth demonstrates atmospheric chemical disequilibrium, that is, a unique cocktail of gases which are present in a highly reactive mixture. No other planet in the solar system enjoys this combination of gases, just as none has the hospitable conditions necessary for life as we know it. Gaia theory states that life itself creates and maintains these seemingly unlikely conditions.

Venus is often called the twin sister of Earth because of its similar size and mass. It may once have had oceans, but with a surface temperature of around 480° C (928° F) — hot enough to melt lead — it is now dry and barren. This is due to the large percentage of carbon dioxide in Venus's atmosphere, which acts like a greenhouse, trapping the intense heat of the Sun. By contrast, Mars is smaller and colder, with a surface temperature averaging -23° C (-9° F), which is tolerable to some forms of life on Earth. Mars also has ice at its poles, though the ice is dry as a result of the high quantities of carbon dioxide in its atmosphere freezing solid. While scientists think that there may be water on Mars, trapped as ice under the surface, this has yet to be proven.

Humankind has been fascinated with the possibility of coming face to face with Martians, and this popular notion was given encouragement by maps of the planet drawn by astronomers that showed straight lines on its surface. One suggestion was that these were canals constructed to carry water from the poles to the desert regions. Space probes in the 1960s and 1970s showed Mars to be a lifeless world, its surface a stony desert frequently ravaged by dust storms.

Flat Earth

Despite the fact that a school of Ancient Greek scholars had empirically shown that the Earth was round, the belief that it was flat persisted until the beginning of the sixteenth century. However, this simplistic belief was not consistent with certain astronomical observations the Greeks made, such as why a star seen in Alexandria failed to appear over Athens. The land surface had to be curved.

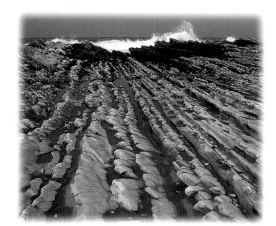

The school of Pythagoras (c.580-500BC) developed the concept of a spherical Earth and its relationship with the rest of the Universe, but made the classic geocentric error of believing that the Sun, Moon, and other planets revolve around us. A few mavericks, notably the Greek astronomer Aristarchus of Samos, challenged this view, suggesting in 250BC that the Earth spins on its axis around the Sun and that its orbital track takes one year to be completed. Unfortunately, Aristarchus was ridiculed for his theories that departed so dramatically from contemporary beliefs.

Nonetheless, the astronomical accuracy of Ancient scholars is breathtaking: in 3BC Greek astronomer and historian Eratosthenes calculated the Earth's circumference to be approximately 40,000 km (24,855 miles) — modern measurements have set it at 40,075 km (24,901 miles) — by studying the different angle of the Sun between two places at noon on Midsummer's Day.

The Ancient Egyptians regarded the Earth as being a flat square, the "base" of a pyramid-shaped sky. In India, early Hindus considered it to be a plate resting on the backs of four elephants standing on a floating turtle. Japanese mythology maintained that the world was originally a watery globe resting on the backbone of an enormous trout. Both Homer and the Greek philosopher Thales of Miletus, living between 800 and 500BC, thought that the Earth was a flat disk floating on water.

From the Dark Ages right up to the seventeenth century, when many Greek discoveries were long forgotten in Europe, the belief that the Earth was flat presided. The Christian church kept tight control on what was or was not "true", to the extent that by studying the Bible, the Archbishop Ussher of Ireland calculated in 1650 that the world was created in 4004BC. He even went as far as to put an exact date and time on the event. By the Middle Ages cartography had become the province of monks whose primary concern was less in presenting geographical accuracy and more in asserting theological ideology. Hence more accurate maps, featuring a spherical globe displayed as a flat map, compiled around AD150 by the Alexandrian scholar Ptolemy, were replaced by those of a flat world restricted to the Mediterranean and surrounding seas, with Jerusalem at the centre. European navigation failed to develop for decades as none but the foolhardy dared venture too far afield, for fear of dropping off the edge. It was Arabic scholars in possession of Ancient Greek geographical knowledge, who helped to change European perceptions. As their people travelled beyond the horizon and lived to tell the tale, European merchants did likewise. A thousand years after it was first written, Ptolemy's work, *Geography*, containing maps, was rediscovered in 1395, thus paving the way for the Great Age of Exploration in the fifteenth and sixteenth centuries. The struggle between Christian ideology and scientific fact continued, the best example being that of Polish polymath Nicolaus Copernicus (1473-1543). He postulated a heliocentric view of the Universe — that the Earth travels around the Sun. In fear of condemnation and retribution by the Roman Catholic church, Copernicus delayed publishing his work for twelve years and died the day he received the first printed copy.

The predominant religious belief of the time was that the Earth was the centre of everything. The work of Copernicus was condemned as heretical and remained banned by the Vatican until 1822. Galileo Galilei (1564-1642), who used the world's first telescope, fared even worse: from his observations of the heavens, he supported Copernicus's revolutionary theories, was put on trial, and found guilty by a Papal Inquisition. Having been forced to deny his discoveries publicly, Galileo spent his final years in exile. It was only in 1992 that the Vatican conceded his work no longer offended Catholic dogma. It is no coincidence that Copernicus's and Galileo's findings were swiftly followed by Newton's mechanistic model. It seems almost as if, having lost the security of geocentrism, humanity's obsession with asserting primacy caused attention to turn to the domination of Nature.

Inaccurate calculations of the circumference of the world caused problems for Christopher Columbus. The Genoese-born explorer (1451-1506) had hoped to find a short sea route to Asia by sailing westward instead of eastward. The globe he used, based on Ptolemy's calculations, showed Japan much nearer than it actually was. This caused the explorer to think he had reached the Indies (Southeast Asia) when in fact he had only got to the Caribbean. Only when Ferdinand Magellan circumnavigated the globe in the early sixteenth century did it become clear that the circumference was larger than previously believed.

The Shifting Continents

The Earth did not always look the way it does now. It is thought that at the time of the Carboniferous period, around 280 million years ago, the land mass on Earth comprised one supercontinent called Pangaea (Greek for "all earth"). This gradually broke into two parts: Laurasia in the north, comprising North America, Greenland, and Eurasia and Gondwana in the south, comprising Australia, South America, Africa, Antarctica, and the Indian subcontinent. Subsequent splits followed, but it was not until 65 million years ago that the world began to look as we know it today, although Australia and Antarctica were still joined.

If you cut out the continents from a contemporary map and piece them together, you will see that they fit rather like a jigsaw. However, in spite of this and Sir Francis Bacon's observation that the east coast of South America appeared as if it had once fitted neatly into the west coast of Africa, scientists thought until recently that the Earth's surface was static. In 1912, when the German professor of meteorology and geophysics Alfred Wegener (1880-1930) first proposed his theory of "continental drift" — that the world's land masses continually drift on the Earth's surface — it was greeted with universal derision. However, as more scientists produced evidence to support Wegener's theory, such as the geophysicists Vine and Matthews and their discoveries of 1963, the concept of plate tectonics developed rapidly.

Plate tectonics theory divides the Earth's lithosphere (crust and upper mantle layer) into a number of large, moveable plates and several smaller ones into which the continents are embedded. This not only explains why rocks found in the Congo match those in Brazil, or why plant and animal distribution is identical across continents separated by vast oceans of water, but also why the Atlantic ocean is 10 metres (33 feet) wider now than it was when Columbus sailed across it. Where two plates push together, mountain ranges are produced. The Himalayas, for example, are believed to have been produced around 45 million years ago, when the Indo-

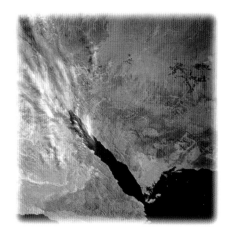

It is hypothesized that oil and coal deposits now mined in the northern hemisphere were actually formed in tropical areas and carried to their present locations by continental drift.

Australian plate moved northward into the Eurasian land mass. When two plates slide sideways against each other this causes earthquakes. The Earth's belt of volcanoes can be charted near the edges of moving plates.

Drawing on this theory of shifting plates we can anticipate what the globe might look like in future. The Americas are moving westward, widening the Atlantic and narrowing the Pacific. The long sliver of west Mexico, between the Pacific and the Gulf of California, is likely to break off and form an island that will float northward. South America, which is moving northward, will compress Central America and Panama. Australia and New Guinea, also drifting northward, will collide with Southeast Asia, and the Mediterranean will dry up as Africa moves north into Europe, creating a new mountain range running from northwest Africa to Turkey. In addition, fragments of East Africa may also split off and drift toward Asia. India, which is still drifting northward, raising the Himalayas, is contributing to the fact that Mount Everest, the world's highest mountain, is becoming taller by at least 25 mm (1 inch) every year and has added 243 mm (8 feet) to its height since the beginning of the twentieth century. Everest is also moving northeastward at a rate of 25 cm (10 inches) every decade.

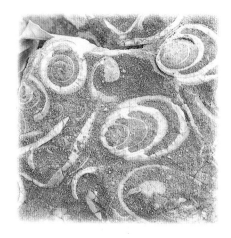

The Changing Landscape

Fossil evidence of sea-dwelling creatures on the tops of mountains illustrates how, when two continental plates collide, mountains are formed from what may have once been an ocean floor. But it is not just these huge tectonic shifts that have changed the face of Earth — at their most dramatic as earthquakes and volcanic activity (see pp.36-7).

All surface rocks are subject to attack by wind, water, ice, frost, and heat. As they are broken into fragments they are washed or blown away to be deposited elsewhere, where they may settle and compact to form new sedimentary deposits (see p.40).

Changes to the Earth's surface are caused by many factors, namely:
* Erosion caused by the weathering of rocks
* The movement of glaciers during the Ice Ages
* Changes in sea level
* Invasions from space in the shape of meteorites
* The impact of civilization

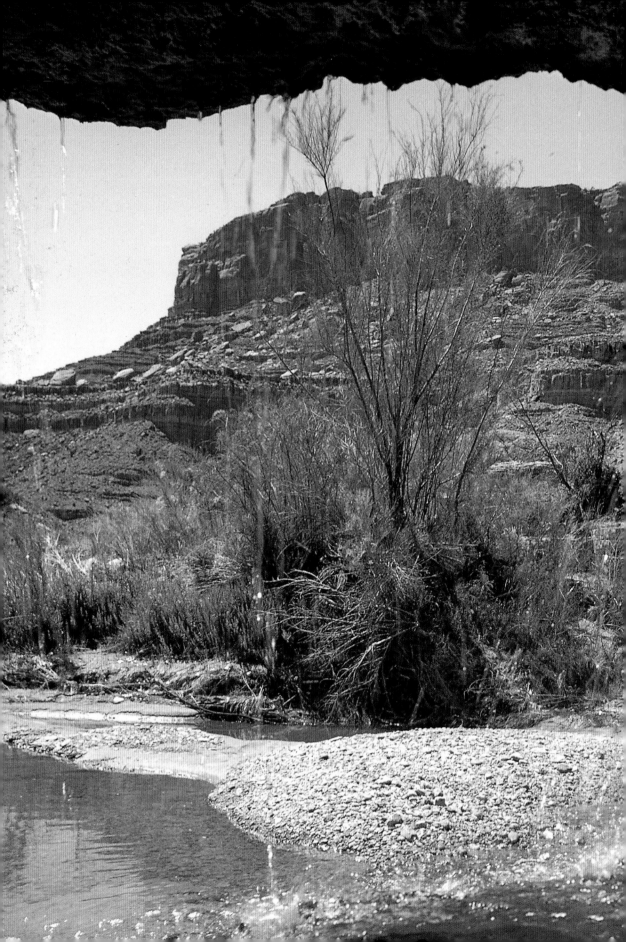

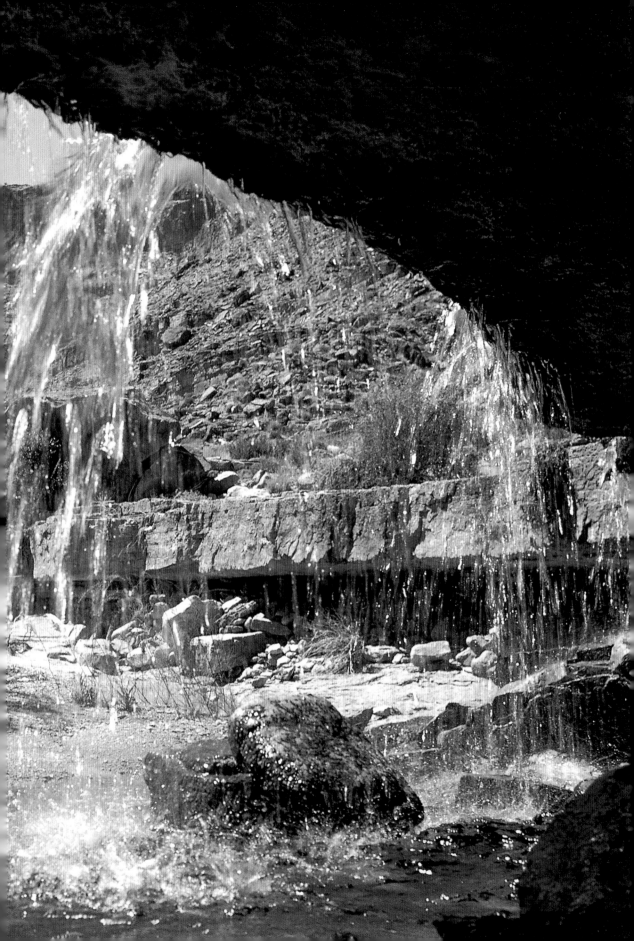

The Grand Canyon in Arizona, USA, offers us the opportunity to see what a slice of the Earth's crust looks like from the inside; its mile-deep rock formations date back 2,000 million years. Scientists believe that the Canyon may have been hollowed out over the last ten million years by the Colorado River. Yet no one has come up with a viable explanation as to what might have happened to the two million million cubic metres of debris that would have been eroded and washed away.

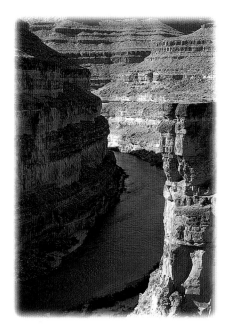

Nowhere is erosion more graphically seen than along coastal areas, where the relentless pounding of the sea eats away at the land, particularly when the rock being eroded is soft, like limestone and chalk. Great Britain, for example, has experienced some dramatic inroads into her coastline: between 1852 and 1897 an area of the Holderness coastline in the northeast of England retreated by an average of 65.5 metres (21 feet), that is, 1.4 metres (4 feet) approximately a year.

Further sculpting of the Earth's landscapes took place during many ice ages. Glaciers, moving at an average of a few inches a day, would have advanced over the land, smoothing down rocks, gouging out valleys, and chiselling down the sides of mountains. The u-shaped fjords of Scandinavia, for example, were produced when glaciers melted. At the end of the last ice age, about ten thousand years ago, the rising sea — which had previously been locked into the polar ice caps, lowering sea levels globally by around 90 metres (295 feet) — engulfed what had previously been land. No longer weighted down by the enormous wedges of ice that covered the land from Scotland to the Thames, northern Britain continues to rise at the expense of its southeastern coastline: London has "sunk" 4.5 metres (15 feet) since Roman times, changing the course of the River Thames. Denmark, northern Germany, and Holland have similarly shifting coastlines.

Space Invaders

The Earth is not just subject to change from within but also from space: fragments of interstellar matter have penetrated our atmosphere and crashed down, scarring the surface of the Earth. The surface of the Moon is pitted in a similar way.

The first globally recognized and largest-known example of a meteor crater, discovered only in 1891, is the Barringer or Meteor Crater in Arizona. It is thought to have been blasted out by a massive piece of nickel and iron 41 metres (1,345 feet) in diameter, weighing something like 300,000 tonnes and travelling at 19 km (12 miles) a second. The near-circular depression is just over 1 km (0.6 miles) in diameter, approximately 175 metres (574 feet) deep, with a rim of up to 48 metres (158 feet) above the surrounding plain.

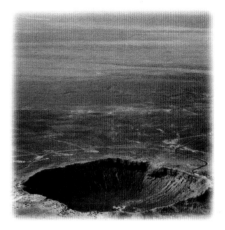

The orthodox scientific community, who insisted that the hole was volcanic in origin, ridiculed the mining entrepreneur, Daniel Moreau Barringer, after whom the crater is named. Barringer was told that evidence of thousands of meteoric fragments near the scene was coincidental. Undeterred, Barringer devoted much of his life and fortune to getting his theory accepted and was finally rewarded in 1930.

Thankfully, because of the vast amount of water on the Earth's surface and the fact that huge swathes of land remain unoccupied, no meteorite has yet crashed on a populated area of this planet. Nonetheless, these space invaders brought with them benefits; in Greenland the Inuits have, for centuries, mined iron deposited by three enormous meteorites. The largest, weighing 34 tonnes, is now in New York's Museum of Natural History.

Humankind has also shaped the land, clearing fens in the Netherlands by pushing back the shoreline or devastating vast tracts to build towns and cities, roads, and transportation networks. The clearing of woodlands in Britain over the centuries has left it relatively forest-free, while depletion of the rainforests in South and Central America continues detrimentally to affect the globe. The following example is a warning of what can happen when the delicate balance of Earth's ecosystems is manipulated.

Desert Swansong

In Roman times there were 600 cities in North Africa, an area known as the "granary of the Roman Empire". Today there is only the aridity of the Sahara Desert covering 8.4 million square kilometres (3.1 million square miles). Desertification is, alarmingly, on the increase, although understanding of the reasons behind it remains incomplete. In the 70 years between 1882 and 1952 the areas of Earth classified as desert rose from 9.4 to 23.3 per cent. In 1984, according to the UN Environmental Programme, 21 million hectares (52 million acres) of land have become nearly or completely useless as the vagaries of weather diminishes rainfall and dries up springs. But the cause of these spreading dust bowls cannot be fully attributed to Nature: indiscriminate deforestation and overgrazing in the interests of logging and agriculture expose the fertile topsoil and allow it to be blown away.

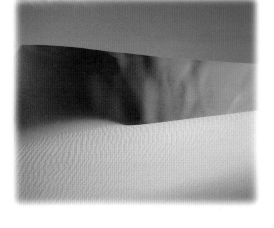

In ancient times the area we now call the Sahara was verdant and productive. Rock paintings, dating from 8000BC, on the walls of ancient caves in Tassili, southern Algeria, reveal pastoral inhabitants tending herds of piebald cattle and hunting gazelles, giraffes, lions, and buffalo. Two thousand years ago the last tribes surrendered to the shifting sands, leaving the increasingly arid and barren land behind. We are not the only generation to have exploited and decimated areas of this planet.

Cosmic Connections

Presented by a flat horizon, it is still hard to imagine that the Earth is spherical. In the same way, it is difficult to conceive that the Earth spins on its axis through space at 1,670 km/h (1,038 miles/h) and orbits around the Sun at 107,280 km/h (66,660 miles/h) — over fifty times faster than Concorde. The Earth completes one turn of its axis every 24 hours and every 365.25 days it circles around the Sun, a distance of 148,800,000 km (9,246,003 miles) every Earth year. However, this has not always been the case: scientists studying growth lines on coral have estimated that some 400 million years ago, when the Earth was spinning faster, thereby producing shorter days, each year was 400 days long.

It is well known that the Earth is subject to the influences of the Sun and the Moon. Not only does the Sun bring life-sustaining heat and light to the planet but it also determines the seasons. In the northern and southern hemispheres these are quite marked, whereas those regions around the equator that are less affected by the angle of the Earth's tilt of 23.5 degrees enjoy more constant climates. Clouds, wind, and rain are all generated by the Sun heating the air, which in turn cools.

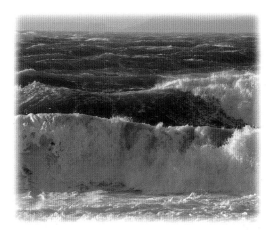

The Sun, and, to a greater extent, the Moon, govern our tides, their gravitational pull on the seas varying according to their relative position to Earth. The highest spring tides occur when the Moon and the Sun are either on the same, or opposite, sides of the Earth and the gravitational pull exerted is at its greatest.

There are many theories about how the Moon came to exist. One, the Big Splash Theory, hypothesizes that the Moon was originally a part of Earth, which broke off when a planet, probably the size of Mars and travelling at speeds over 16,000 km/h (9,942 miles/h), came crashing into her. Circling the Earth and spinning on its own axis, the Moon's cycle lasts 27 days, though we only ever see one side of it. The dark side of the Moon was first viewed in 1959 when the Russian spacecraft Luna 3 flew behind it.

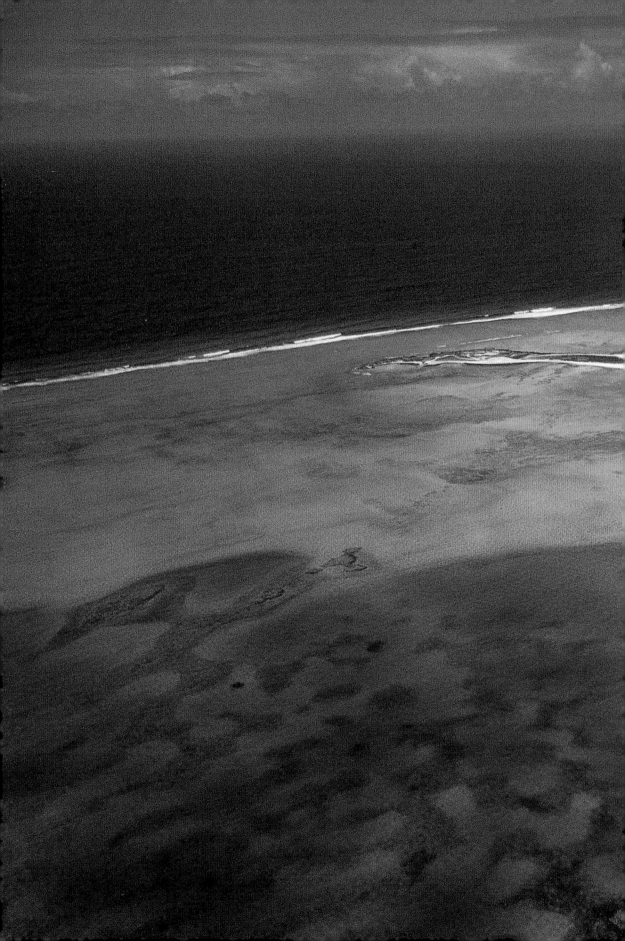

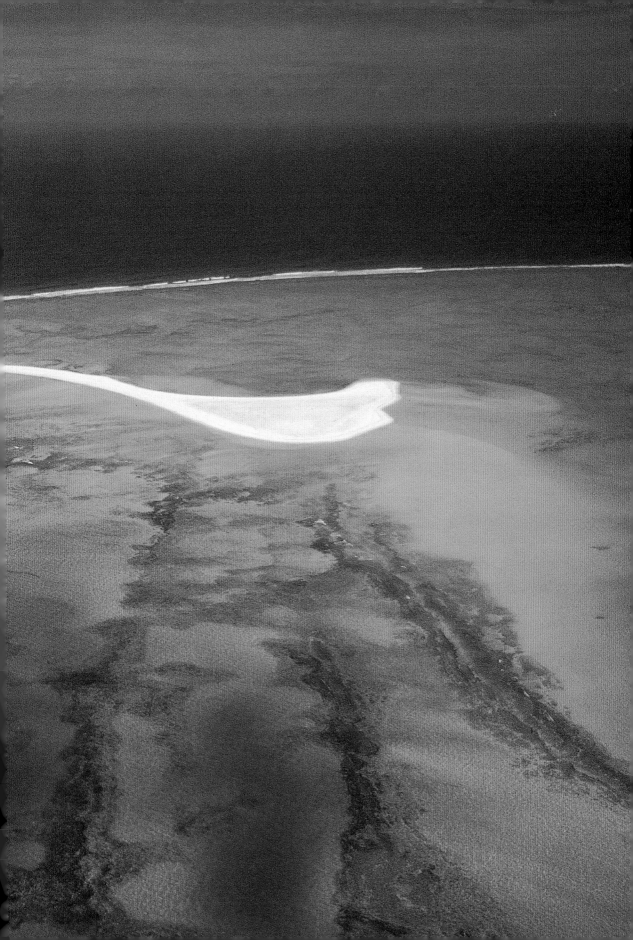

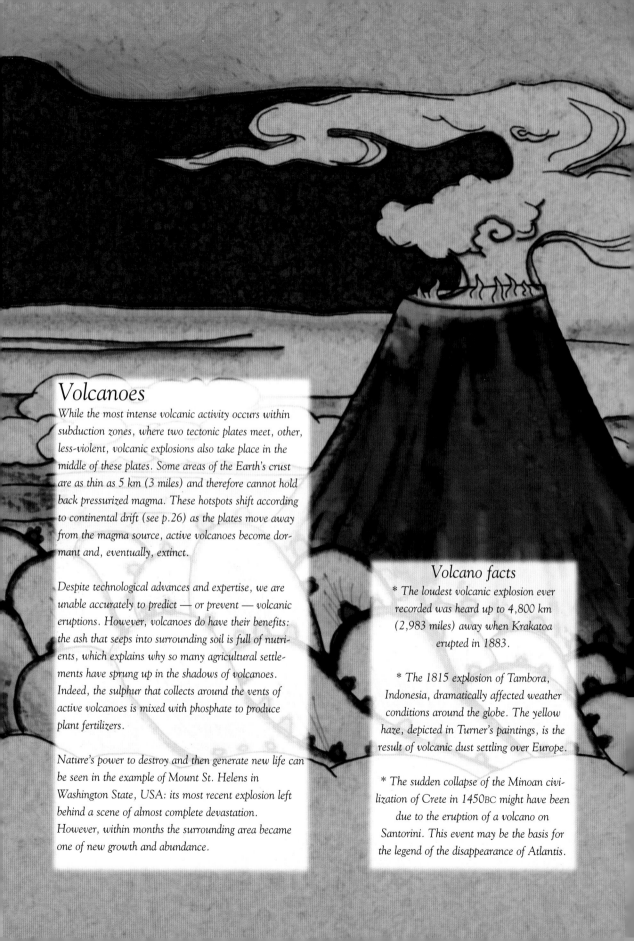

Volcanoes

While the most intense volcanic activity occurs within subduction zones, where two tectonic plates meet, other, less-violent, volcanic explosions also take place in the middle of these plates. Some areas of the Earth's crust are as thin as 5 km (3 miles) and therefore cannot hold back pressurized magma. These hotspots shift according to continental drift (see p.26) as the plates move away from the magma source, active volcanoes become dormant and, eventually, extinct.

Despite technological advances and expertise, we are unable accurately to predict — or prevent — volcanic eruptions. However, volcanoes do have their benefits: the ash that seeps into surrounding soil is full of nutrients, which explains why so many agricultural settlements have sprung up in the shadows of volcanoes. Indeed, the sulphur that collects around the vents of active volcanoes is mixed with phosphate to produce plant fertilizers.

Nature's power to destroy and then generate new life can be seen in the example of Mount St. Helens in Washington State, USA: its most recent explosion left behind a scene of almost complete devastation. However, within months the surrounding area became one of new growth and abundance.

Volcano facts

* The loudest volcanic explosion ever recorded was heard up to 4,800 km (2,983 miles) away when Krakatoa erupted in 1883.

* The 1815 explosion of Tambora, Indonesia, dramatically affected weather conditions around the globe. The yellow haze, depicted in Turner's paintings, is the result of volcanic dust settling over Europe.

* The sudden collapse of the Minoan civilization of Crete in 1450BC might have been due to the eruption of a volcano on Santorini. This event may be the basis for the legend of the disappearance of Atlantis.

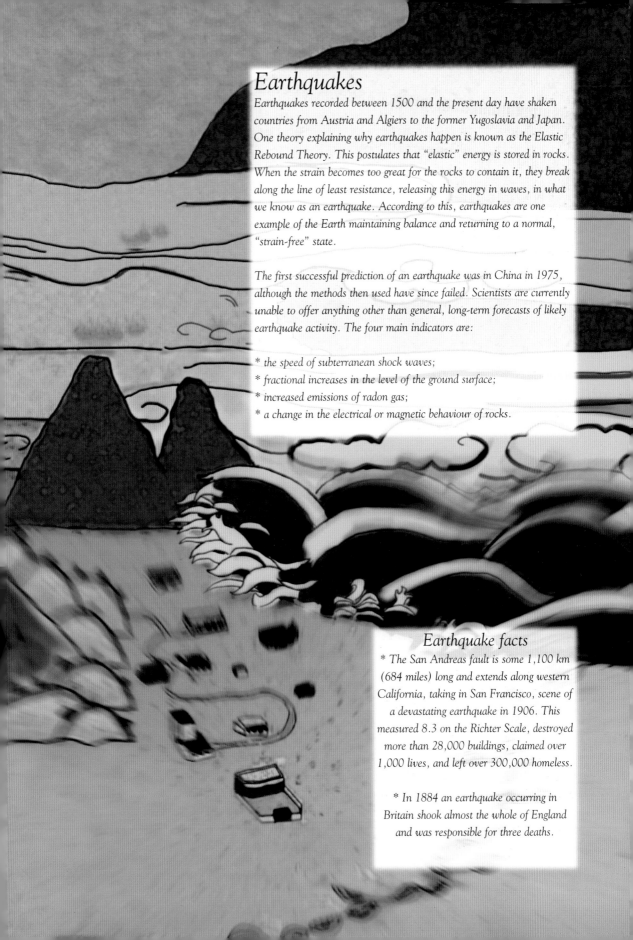

Earthquakes

Earthquakes recorded between 1500 and the present day have shaken countries from Austria and Algiers to the former Yugoslavia and Japan. One theory explaining why earthquakes happen is known as the Elastic Rebound Theory. This postulates that "elastic" energy is stored in rocks. When the strain becomes too great for the rocks to contain it, they break along the line of least resistance, releasing this energy in waves, in what we know as an earthquake. According to this, earthquakes are one example of the Earth maintaining balance and returning to a normal, "strain-free" state.

The first successful prediction of an earthquake was in China in 1975, although the methods then used have since failed. Scientists are currently unable to offer anything other than general, long-term forecasts of likely earthquake activity. The four main indicators are:

* the speed of subterranean shock waves;
* fractional increases in the level of the ground surface;
* increased emissions of radon gas;
* a change in the electrical or magnetic behaviour of rocks.

Earthquake facts

* The San Andreas fault is some 1,100 km (684 miles) long and extends along western California, taking in San Francisco, scene of a devastating earthquake in 1906. This measured 8.3 on the Richter Scale, destroyed more than 28,000 buildings, claimed over 1,000 lives, and left over 300,000 homeless.

* In 1884 an earthquake occurring in Britain shook almost the whole of England and was responsible for three deaths.

Geothermal Benefits

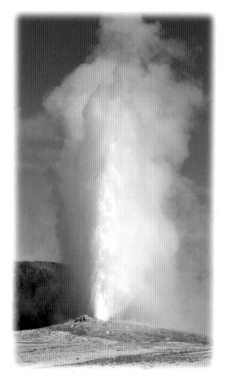

The Earth's core acts like a gigantic nuclear reactor, with intense heat constantly radiating upward from the decay of radioactive material such as uranium. This vast energy reserve remains largely unexploited, despite being cheap, reliable, and near pollution-free. Just as you would find if you pulled a piece of unbaked dough apart by the edges, crustal plates pulled away from each other by continental drift produce a thin, weak area in some places. Apart from these being the sites of hot spot volcanoes, these separating plates allow molten magma to rise, heating any underground water, which then erupts as hot springs, or "geysers" — an old Norse word meaning "to gush".

Iceland, which has more geysers than anywhere else in the world, uses this geothermal energy to supply hot water and heating to homes and commercial enterprises. By 1980, 70 per cent of houses in Iceland were heated by geothermal energy. However, it is also a significant source of power in New Zealand, the Philippines, California, and Mexico. Geysers in northern California, for example, can satisfy most of the electrical energy needs of San Francisco. And in Russia and Iceland, where the climate inhibits normal vegetation growth, geothermally heated greenhouses force crops on. In Iceland waste geothermally heated water filling lagoons allows bathers to enjoy heated outdoor swimming pools, despite freezing ambient temperatures.

Even where there are no naturally occurring hot springs, water pumped to the dry, hot rocks beneath the Earth's surface can produce enough steam to generate electricity and drive turbines. While some geothermal power stations have been built over this natural source of energy, in the vast majority of cases the supply is drilled and piped to wherever it is going to be utilized.

As fossil fuels continue to be depleted and environmentalists are warning people of the dangers of nuclear energy, an increasing number of countries are investigating geothermal energy and its potential to power our needs.

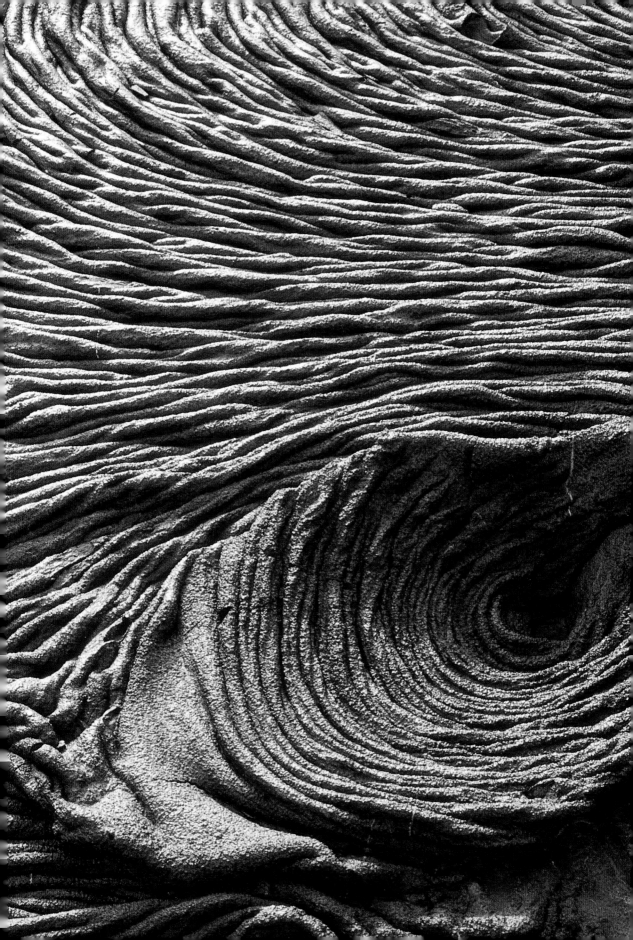

A Window On The Past

The Earth's crust is made up of little more than half a dozen different minerals that are formed into rocks in one of three ways. Each of their names describes the process:

Igneous

(from the Latin, igneus, meaning "fiery")
Once molten material, or magma, igneous rocks are either pushed to the surface, where they cool and harden to form fine-grained, glass-like extrusive rocks, or which solidify underground, producing coarse-grained rocks, called "intrusive". All igneous rocks are crystalline. Examples include feldspar, granite, basalt, syenite, and rhyolite.

Sedimentary

(from the Latin sedimentum — settling)
Sedimentary rocks are formed over millennia as fragments of rock and bony remains of animals accumulate and are compressed to form sedimentary deposits. Examples include sandstone, limestone, gravel, sand, silt, clays, coal, shale, and chalk, many of which are used as building materials.

Metamorphic

(from the Greek, metamorphosis, meaning "changed from")
Under particular conditions of heat and pressure, existing sedimentary and igneous rocks can change their chemical and, therefore, physical composition and be "metamorphosed" into a different type of rock. Marble is a limestone that has been changed in this way. Other examples include schist, gneiss, and slate.

Rocks and the remains of plants and creatures compressed in them enable scientists to build up a picture of the Earth's history, and that of her inhabitants, over billions of years. Before radiocarbon dating was developed by American physicist Willard F. Libby in the mid-1950s, archaeologists and geologists conducted their studies through painstaking examination of soil and rock layering. While observation, as with the dating of tree rings, can be less accurate, the atomic data accumulated from radiocarbon dating gets progressively more difficult to detect, so this method cannot be used reliably for remains older than 35,000 years.

The climate and vegetation of a particular area can be accurately "unearthed" by examining something as tiny as fossilized pollen grains: pollen analysis conducted in Israel in 1987 revealed that inhabitants living close to the Sea of Galilee 5,000 years ago cleared away oak forests to grow olive trees for food and oil; when this production declined in the third century AD so too did the number of trees.

Ancient rocks also hold within them the story of Earth's vulnerability to external attack. Paleomagnetism — or the study of the magnetic field of the mineral content of rocks — has revealed that, as magma from volcanoes cools to form igneous rocks, minerals within acquire and retain a magnetic quality and thus lie in the direction of the magnetic north at the time. The complete displacement of the outer shell of the Earth has caused a reversal of the north and south poles at least 170 times in the past 100 million years, and ten times within the past three million, that is, within the time that civilization has existed. It is not so much continental drift (see p.26) as "crustal shift". This means that a compass that once pointed north would now point south.

Evidence of reversed polarity in rocks can therefore shed light on the catastrophic events that have been documented in stories such as the Babylonian epic *Gilgamesh*, on which the biblical story of Noah's Flood is based. It may also account for the legend of the disappearance of Atlantis, to which Plato referred in *Timaeus* and *Critias*, as lying west of the Straits of Gibraltar. While many researchers argue that Atlantis did exist — and by ingenious reasoning try to prove it — it is more likely to be an allegorical tale linking many different accounts about the end of various cultures during one or more pole reversals.

The effects of alteration of the Earth's speed and angle of rotation would be catastrophic: oceans would be displaced, giant tidal waves would engulf vast tracts of land; global earthquakes, dramatic climactic and temperature changes would seize the Earth. All of these have been explained mythologically by ancient peoples from the Native American Hopis and the pre-Columbian Maya, to the Selungs of Burma and the Somali of Africa. In a papyrus now in safe-keeping in St. Petersburg, Russia, Ancient Egyptians describe a cataclysm that "turned the world upside down".

Some researchers believe that no terrestrial activity is violent enough to be capable of producing this type of destruction on such a massive scale. They postulate that pole shifts have been caused by the close promixity of an enormous celestial body, possibly a planet like Venus. Recorded experiences of our early ancestors reveal that they believed this to be fact rather than fiction. However, Charles Hapgood, author of *Earth's Shifting Crust*, suggests that the trigger for a crustal slip is more likely to be the imbalance of the polar ice masses, increasing the natural "wobble" of the Earth as it rotates — not unlike the action of an unbalanced washing machine load.

The last cataclysm is estimated to have taken place around 10,000 years ago. This would account for the discovery of animals in Alaska and Siberia that were literally frozen in mid-action and the instant extinction of life. No one knows when such a catastrophe might happen again.

Soil is the vital material on which humankind relies for growing food. Soil is a mixture of eroded rocks, decayed plants, and rotted animals, within which pockets of air and water offer a home to countless bacteria, fungi, tiny plants, and animals. It is estimated that there are more living organisms in the soil than in the whole of Earth's other environments put together. However, its fertility and ability to hold or repel water varies with its chemical composition. Clay and peat, for example, are rich in nutrients, but while the former is heavy and does not allow water to pass through, the latter retains a large amount of water and is very spongy and boggy in texture. By contrast, neither sandy nor chalky soils are high in nutrients and therefore are less fertile. However, both offer good drainage for the plants that do grow in them.

Magnetic Earth

While it is commonly thought that orthodox science provides an answer to just about everything, there are many natural phenomena that remain unaccounted for. In some areas scientific explanations of certain process-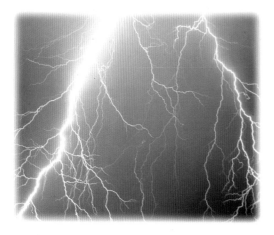es of life have been found only recently, although the understanding and use of them by ancient peoples goes back many hundreds of years. For example, although geomagnetism — the fact that the Earth behaves like a giant magnet — was first demonstrated only in the seventeenth century, early compasses, using crystal magnetite — or lodestone — date back to the Vikings. It is still not fully understood how the Earth's electromagnetism is generated by the molten metal at its outer core, but the outer core of the Earth is thought to generate temperatures in excess of 4,000° C (8,480° F) and magnets usually stop working when they get very hot. One hypothesis, called Dynamic Theory, suggests that the convection currents within this molten metal act like wires in a dynamo.

All matter, including that of the human body, is both electric and magnetic. But, again, the relationship between these two fundamental forces was only discovered in the nineteenth century by Scottish physicist James Clerk Maxwell (1831-79). All our body's biochemical exchanges are underpinned by electricity and medical researchers measure these currents in the brain and heart using electroencephalograms and electrocardiograms (EEG and ECG). Our skin also demonstrates electrodermal activity and under certain conditions, such as walking on a dry nylon carpet, for example, individuals have been found — harmlessly — to build up electrostatic charges of up to 20,000-30,000 volts. This is why we sometimes get a "shock" from shaking someone's hand or when touching a car door. The electrical nature of humankind — and hence of life itself — is graphically portrayed in Michaelangelo's painting of God and Man touching fingertips on the ceiling of the Sistine Chapel and was the basis of Mary Shelley's story of Frankenstein's monster.

While those in authority prefer to keep such knowledge under wraps, we are indubitably affected by electrical and electronic equipment such as overhead power cables, mobile phones, visual display units, and underground cables and we have probably yet to experience the full extent of their detrimental effects. Illnesses thought to stem from our interaction with such equipment ranges from headaches and insomnia to leukaemia and blackouts. One researcher found that there was a 40 per cent increase in suicide cases in areas with high electromagnetic fields caused by man-made equipment. And increased magnetic and electrical exposure in laboratory animals has been thought to be responsible for chromosome abnormalities. However, the effects are not all negative and certain rhythmically pulsating magnetic fields can be beneficial to the body's ability to regenerate itself.

Given that the Earth's electromagnetic radiation is affected by factors such as the type of minerals in the rocks, subterranean water, and the existence of man-made structures should we be so surprised that we are affected biologically and psychologically by the intangible processes constantly going on in and around our Earth? Jung referred to this as "psychic localization" — the ability of some, highly sensitive, individuals in certain places in the world to experience altered states of consciousness and hence tap in to the harmonizing influences of the natural world. Could this be why some potent spots around the globe are known as "sacred places" (see also pp.90-1)?

In Chapter Two, *Sacred Earth*, we take a look at the electromagnetism, or "subtle energy", of human beings, animals, and birds, and how this affects, and is affected by, the Earth's radiation.

Natural mysteries

* *El Niño: the periodic, abnormal oceanic warming within the Pacific has a detrimental economic, as well as an environmental effect, since the cold nutrient-rich currents that boost the fishing industry are changed by it. This unpredictable and little-understood natural phenomenon also upsets established dry weather patterns, causing rains and floods that wash away topsoil, affecting subsequent harvests.*

* *Cameroon killer lakes: in the 1980s, thousands of people died mysteriously near Lake Nyos in the Cameroon highlands of West Africa. A scientific expedition later found that the cause was a lethal concentration of carbon dioxide gas stored underground for thousands of years, which had seeped up to the surface. This burst not only asphyxiated the surrounding populace and their cattle but also destroyed large areas of vegetation.*

* *The weather has long been known to affect health. Damp conditions can cause joint pains and immobility, particularly among arthritics and rheumatics. Before a thunderstorm some people have a tendency to suffer headaches due to the positive ionization of the atmosphere. In some parts of Europe the Föhn wind is believed to be the catalyst for mood changes, migraines, insomnia, and anxiety.*

* *Atmospheric ions are known to affect serotonin levels, which can either cause depression and irritability or serenity and calmness.*

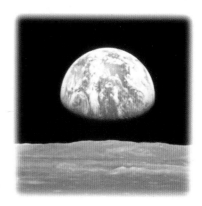

Sacred Earth

Despite the Earth's land masses having separated long before human beings walked on them, there are remarkable similarities between the creation myths of cultures separated by both time and distance. The import of these tales lies beyond their great appeal to the imagination of story-telling: they illustrate universal archetypes that tap in to our collective psychological need to understand the whys and wherefores of the human condition and our inter-relationship with Earth. While today we turn to scientific technology to explain how life on Earth began, early civilizations wove their suppositions into stories. The similarities between these myths across a range and diversity of cultures demonstrate the universal nature of many age-old questions and the answers to them that flow from our collective unconscious.

Myths and Science

Ancient Chinese mythology, accounting for the creation of the Universe, speaks of an egg-shaped ocean of chaos containing the complementary forces of yin and yang, which variously represent negative and positive, feminine and masculine, darkness and light. According to legend the "warring energies" inside this cosmic egg exploded, causing dense elements to form the Earth and the lighter ones to form the sky. This 4,000-year-old

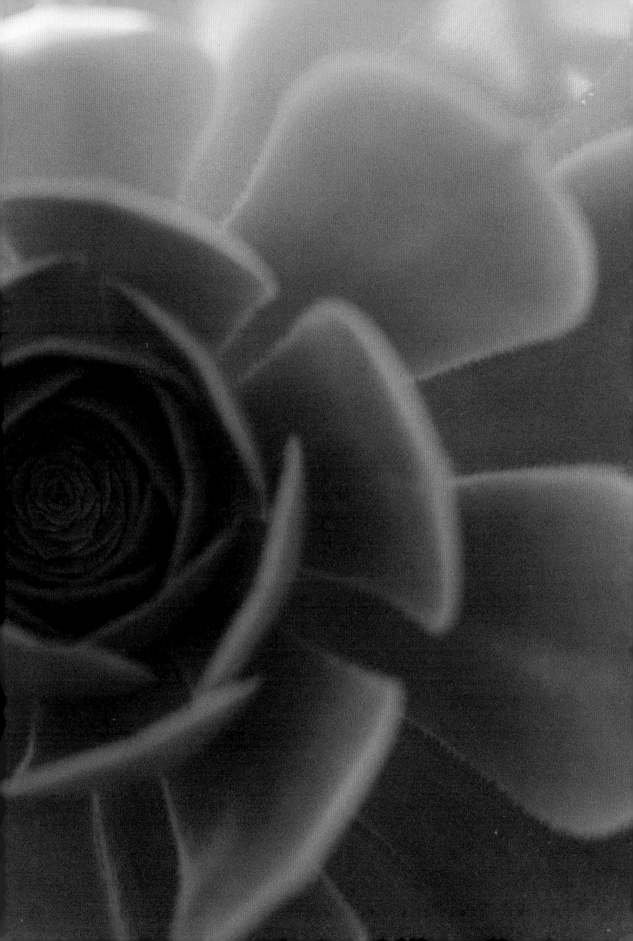

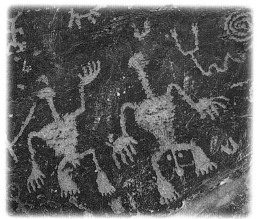

myth seems no more fanciful than the Big Bang Theory, which was hypothesized only in the twentieth century. Similarly, the Greek writer Hesiod, in his *Theogony*, or *Birth of the Gods*, 700BC, relates how Chaos gave birth to Gaia (Earth), Tartarus (the underworld), and Eros (Love). This could represent life in its triplicity of body, mind, and spirit: the conscious in the form of the physical Earth; the subconscious as the underworld; and the superconscious represented by the concept of love. While the conscious and subconscious are well represented by scientific endeavours, there remains an expanding, "bizarre" form of cosmic energy that continues to puzzle contemporary cosmologists. In the light of Hesiod's work, perhaps this energy can be explained by the third of Chaos's creations, love.

Mythological stories of deities remain compelling, appealing to our innermost selves by expressing universal themes or models of experience that represent the spiritual wisdom of countless generations. Their richly symbolic language allows each individual flexibility of interpretation, often hinting at an innate knowledge that orthodox science leaves largely to the realms of philosophy and religion. For example, a number of creation myths, reminiscent of the Bible story of Adam and Eve, speak of humans having been created by a divine being from Earth's raw materials (see right).

Clay and DNA

The Ainu of Japan also talk of their creator god, Kamui, moulding the first humans from earth, using sticks of willow for their spines. In the Middle East, Ancient Mesopotamian and Sumerian cultures (where females were considered equal to males) believed that their goddesses of creation each spat on a lump of clay to make human life. The Hopi tribe of Arizona believe that two brothers descended from heaven and used clay to make human beings, endowing them with life through ritual chanting. Apart from the primordial soup theory, some scientists hypothesize that inorganic, self-replicating crystals of clay were the template from which complex, organic molecules such as RNA and DNA were formed.

In addition to offering explanations for deep philosophical conundrums, archetypal stories reflect everyday human conflicts, such as the battle between good and evil. They also inform us — indeed, attempt to justify — the dominant view of the time, particularly with regard to concepts such as power and leadership, including the relationship between men and women. In patriarchal philosophies a male god inevitably is the creator of the Earth, first creating man and then as a mate or "helper", woman. The relative status of the sexes also becomes apparent from a culture's mythology. In Ancient Greece, one of the world's major early patriarchal civilizations, the supremacy of Gaia (see p.48), a legacy of earlier, more peaceful, nature-loving, and matrifocal civilizations, was overshadowed first by her son Cronus, and then his son, Zeus. The mythology of Ancient Greece and its subsequent dethronement of the Mother Goddess and suppression of goddess culture, can be linked historically with the emerging authority of masculine principles, emphasizing war and sexual dominance. This was brought on by the invasion of peaceful, art-loving cultures of Old Europe by patrifocal, warring Indo-European peoples. Hence stories emerged recanting the humiliation of Hera by her unfaithful husband, Zeus; the rape of Demeter by Poseidon; and the forcible abduction of Persephone by Hades.

The worship of Gaia, which had mainly centred around Attica from 1500BC, fell away even more dramatically after AD400, when the patriarchal Hebrew, Christian, and later Muslim religions dominated the known world. As the female goddesses of pagan cultures faded in prominence, there was an accompanying lessening of the power and influence of women in society.

Genesis 2:7 tells us: "And the Lord God formed man of the dust of the ground and breathed into his nostrils the breath of life; and man became a living soul."
This is a wonderful explanation of the intrinsic physical and spiritual nature of humanity. We are then told that God removed a rib from Adam to create woman, Eve. This story is almost identical to one in Siberian mythology, in which man is created from mud around a stony skeleton, and woman is produced from his rib.

According to the Native American Modoc, the creator god, Kumush, could bring a man back to life from only a single hair. Could early mythology have been hinting at an advanced science capable of modern cloning? Cloning, the production of a genetically identical twin, has been made possible by the knowledge that each human cell contains a nucleus that holds the unique genetic blueprint for a particular individual. In theory, one could clone a dead person from just one hair. The legend of Modoc is perhaps less a case of resurrection and more one of cloning.

Gaia the Mother Goddess

Hesiod tells us that the female, "deep-breasted Earth"
goddess, Gaia, appeared out of Chaos and gave birth to
a son, Ouranos, more commonly known as Uranus, the
starlit sky. Gaia then mated with Uranus to produce the
"ancestors of humankind", the Titans.

Many cultures wove similar stories around the symbolic
mating of the Earth and sky. For some, such as the
Ancient Greek or Maori deities, the Earth is always
female and the sky male. Others depict a male Earth god
and female sky goddess, such as Geb and Nut in
Egyptian mythology.

Each of the deities produced by Gaia, Uranus, and their
progeny, serves to symbolize either the various forces of
Nature or abstract human qualities. For example, after
producing six male and six female Titans, including the
youngest son Cronus, Gaia bore the Cyclopes, the one-
eyed storm deities representing thunder, lightning, and
thunderbolts.

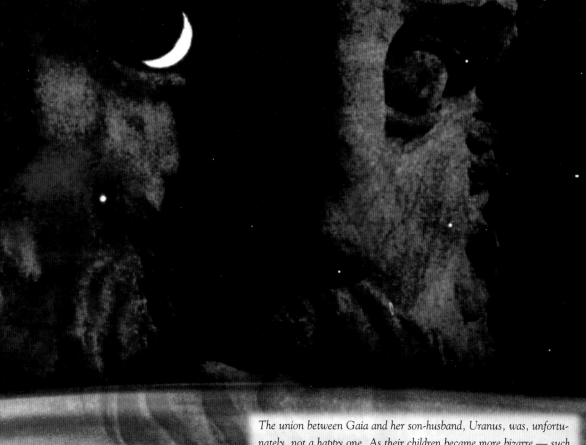

The union between Gaia and her son-husband, Uranus, was, unfortunately, not a happy one. As their children became more bizarre — such as the 100-armed, 50-headed Centimanes — Uranus buried each of them at birth back into her body.

Angry and humiliated, Gaia finally persuaded Cronus, the youngest Titan and personification of Time, to exact revenge on his father. Cronus castrated Uranus, tossing his genitals into the sea from which — somewhat ironically — young Aphrodite, the Goddess of Love and Beauty was born.

Cronus became the most powerful male god and fathered, with his Titan sister Rhea, a new dynasty of Zeus (the sky), Poseidon (the sea), Hades (the underworld), Hestia (goddess of hearth and temple), Demeter (goddess of grain, who succeeded Gaia as the representation of nature), and Hera (goddess of marriage).

However, history soon repeated itself as Cronus attempted to eliminate each one of his children by swallowing them whole. Gaia and Rhea hatched a plan whereby Cronus thought that he was swallowing the youngest, Zeus, when it was actually a stone wrapped in baby's clothing. Later, Zeus defeated Cronus, tricking him into regurgitating his siblings, and became the promiscuous, philandering chief god, ruler of Heaven and Earth.

The Gaia Hypothesis

In 1972, an independent scientist-philosopher, James Lovelock, coined the term "Gaia theory" for his hypothesis that planet Earth is alive and is a self-regulating ecosystem in its own right, which can become sick. Gaia theory identifies some of the commonly observed characteristics that living organisms, such as mammals, share with the Earth — including metabolism, evolution, self-healing, and thermostasis. Lovelock set about taking Earth through a rigorous health check in order to highlight its vulnerable state and the extent to which she is infected by "people plague".

Masculine and Feminine

Humankind across many cultures seems to be more comfortable with a separation of genders, rather than their integration — which may account for men finding it so difficult to acknowledge their "feminine" side and for women feeling uncomfortable with their "masculine" traits. Patriarchal theologies such as Christianity continue to perceive the Divinity as male. Assigning God with a gender may have begun as a way of identifying with a concept that otherwise would be totally alien to the human mind. Nonetheless, over the centuries this has often been exploited as a means of subjugating the female gender. The animistic view of traditional, indigenous societies regarded the Universe and everything in it as being alive, hence inanimate objects, such as rocks, were deemed to have human qualities. This spiritual appreciation of the environment encouraged humans to live in harmony with natural surroundings, whereas more recent materialistic cultures view the natural world as merely a resource to be exploited for the good of humankind, regardless of the cost.

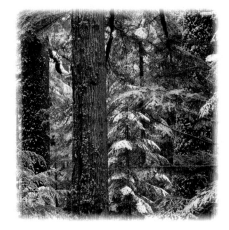

Despite the individual practices of the different traditions found within it, paganism offers a flexible approach to spirituality by respecting individual beliefs and unique needs. In the same way that Buddhists believe in "right livelihood", pagan ethics state that "If it harms none, do what you will". All that is required is to respect and hold sacred the natural world, our fellow creatures, and humankind.

While we may not consider ourselves pagans as such, few of us remain untouched by their practices: both Hallowe'en and Yuletide (or Christmas) are pagan festivals and customs such as "beating the bounds" and "apple bobbing" are carried out annually by pagans and Christians alike.

Seventeenth-century mystic, Jakob Boehme (1575-1624), challenged the notion of a male creator when he suggested that God was androgynous, basing his theory on what he viewed to be the hermaphroditic Adam "giving birth" to Eve. Boehme argued that, since God created Man in His own image our creator must also be androgynous. This view reflects earlier widespread beliefs in an androgynous primordial being that is both all things and, because opposite polarities cancel each other out, nothing. It is only when this hermaphroditic being embarks on the act of creation that the products — such as a female Earth and a male sky, or vice versa — result in the splitting of feminine and masculine characteristics. The concept of the division of the male and female souls, however, does not always require the domination of one over the other. This is demonstrated by the world's oldest form of religion, one that has no messiah, saints, founders, or leaders, and is arguably one of the world's fastest-growing Western spiritual movements: paganism.

The Old Religion

The term paganism comes from the Latin, *pagus*, meaning "village", originally referring to a country-dweller, who were thought of as respecting the environment and recognizing harmony in Nature. When monotheistic religions took hold, the word pagan began to carry derogatory associations. In an age when "green" issues are becoming increasingly important, paganism is enjoying a revival. For many, celebrating several deities does not mean abandoning one god, as each deity is acknowledged as a different aspect of the Divine.

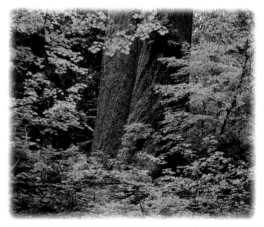

Paganism has particular appeal for women: goddesses have equal status with gods, so female worshippers have never been disenfranchized. The goddess plays a vital role, demonstrating key values of conservation and nurturing, whereas in paternalistic, monotheistic religions the feminine principle is secondary. However, these female deities are not restricted to the softer arts of love, marriage, beauty, and fertility, but are patronesses of all human endeavours — including war and magic.

Pagan deities are different from those of monotheistic religions in that they take on attributes which many might consider feminine. In English folklore, the Green Man, frequently depicted as a head covered in vegetation, symbolizes the secret laws of Nature, including the land's return to fertility after winter. These Natural Laws are principles that enable pagans to live in harmony with the environment. The reverence of the leafy elements of the Green Man is in keeping with modern understanding of the importance of leaves in regulating the Earth's ecosystem and creating and maintaining a life-giving atmosphere. When we explore the similarities between our bodies and the body of Earth, we will see that leaves represent the planet's lungs.

Pagans honour a plethora of gods and goddesses and are pantheistic — regarding the Divine to be everywhere and in everything, animate or inanimate. While entities such as animals, trees, and rocks are not worshipped in the same sense that the monotheistic religions worship God, they are revered as manifesting the Divine Spirit. Pagan deities are considered to inhabit special places, such as groves of trees. This is why pagan festivals are held outdoors, where humans can celebrate their close connection with Nature.

Pagans intuitively understand the delicate, dynamic inter-relationship not only between humankind and the environment but also between the many regulatory processes that Gaia juggles so effectively.

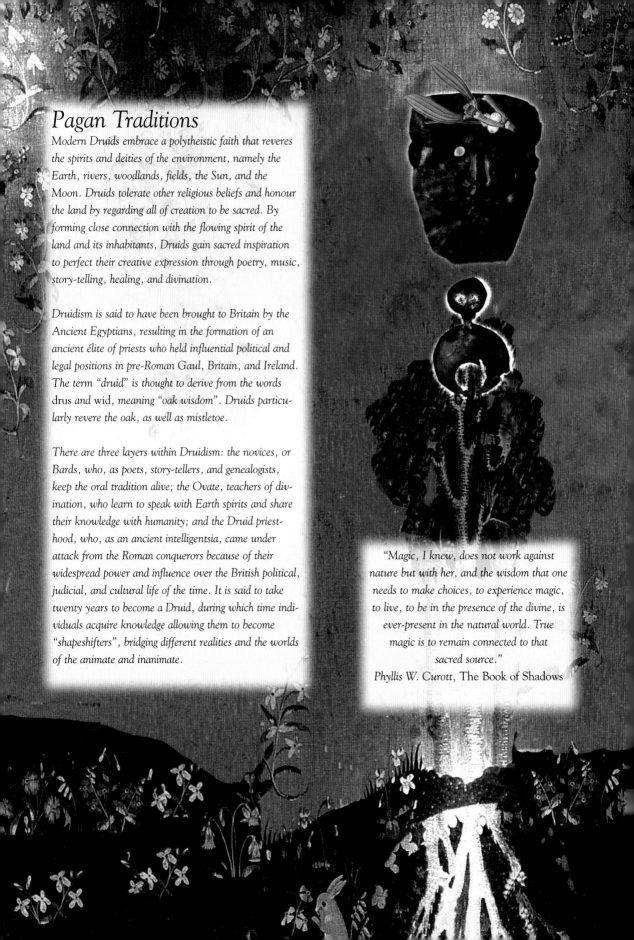

Pagan Traditions

Modern Druids embrace a polytheistic faith that reveres the spirits and deities of the environment, namely the Earth, rivers, woodlands, fields, the Sun, and the Moon. Druids tolerate other religious beliefs and honour the land by regarding all of creation to be sacred. By forming close connection with the flowing spirit of the land and its inhabitants, Druids gain sacred inspiration to perfect their creative expression through poetry, music, story-telling, healing, and divination.

Druidism is said to have been brought to Britain by the Ancient Egyptians, resulting in the formation of an ancient élite of priests who held influential political and legal positions in pre-Roman Gaul, Britain, and Ireland. The term "druid" is thought to derive from the words drus and wid, meaning "oak wisdom". Druids particularly revere the oak, as well as mistletoe.

There are three layers within Druidism: the novices, or Bards, who, as poets, story-tellers, and genealogists, keep the oral tradition alive; the Ovate, teachers of divination, who learn to speak with Earth spirits and share their knowledge with humanity; and the Druid priesthood, who, as an ancient intelligentsia, came under attack from the Roman conquerors because of their widespread power and influence over the British political, judicial, and cultural life of the time. It is said to take twenty years to become a Druid, during which time individuals acquire knowledge allowing them to become "shapeshifters", bridging different realities and the worlds of the animate and inanimate.

"Magic, I knew, does not work against nature but with her, and the wisdom that one needs to make choices, to experience magic, to live, to be in the presence of the divine, is ever-present in the natural world. True magic is to remain connected to that sacred source."

Phyllis W. Curott, The Book of Shadows

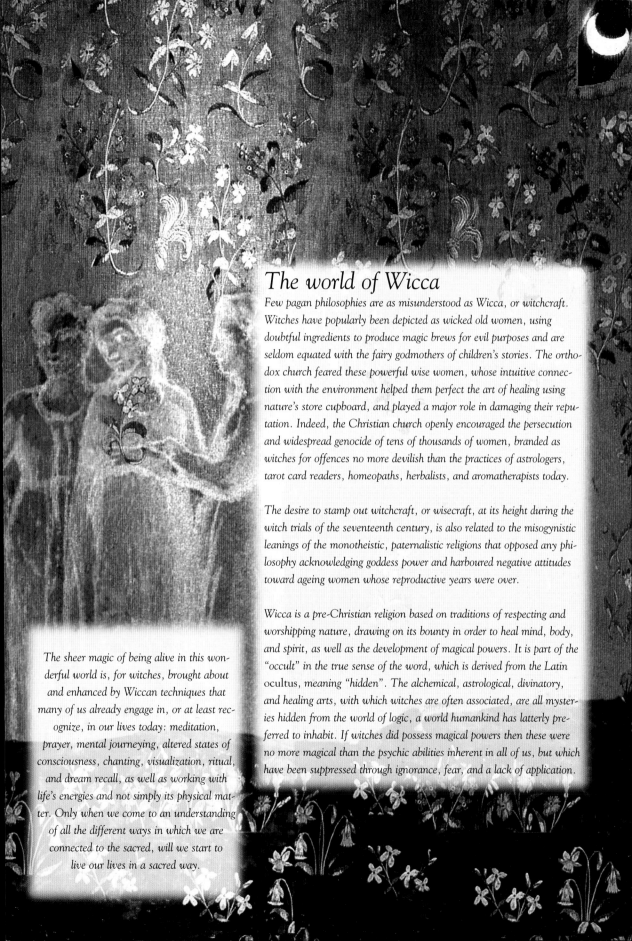

The world of Wicca

Few pagan philosophies are as misunderstood as Wicca, or witchcraft. Witches have popularly been depicted as wicked old women, using doubtful ingredients to produce magic brews for evil purposes and are seldom equated with the fairy godmothers of children's stories. The orthodox church feared these powerful wise women, whose intuitive connection with the environment helped them perfect the art of healing using nature's store cupboard, and played a major role in damaging their reputation. Indeed, the Christian church openly encouraged the persecution and widespread genocide of tens of thousands of women, branded as witches for offences no more devilish than the practices of astrologers, tarot card readers, homeopaths, herbalists, and aromatherapists today.

The desire to stamp out witchcraft, or wisecraft, at its height during the witch trials of the seventeenth century, is also related to the misogynistic leanings of the monotheistic, paternalistic religions that opposed any philosophy acknowledging goddess power and harboured negative attitudes toward ageing women whose reproductive years were over.

Wicca is a pre-Christian religion based on traditions of respecting and worshipping nature, drawing on its bounty in order to heal mind, body, and spirit, as well as the development of magical powers. It is part of the "occult" in the true sense of the word, which is derived from the Latin ocultus, meaning "hidden". The alchemical, astrological, divinatory, and healing arts, with which witches are often associated, are all mysteries hidden from the world of logic, a world humankind has latterly preferred to inhabit. If witches did possess magical powers then these were no more magical than the psychic abilities inherent in all of us, but which have been suppressed through ignorance, fear, and a lack of application.

The sheer magic of being alive in this wonderful world is, for witches, brought about and enhanced by Wiccan techniques that many of us already engage in, or at least recognize, in our lives today: meditation, prayer, mental journeying, altered states of consciousness, chanting, visualization, ritual, and dream recall, as well as working with life's energies and not simply its physical matter. Only when we come to an understanding of all the different ways in which we are connected to the sacred, will we start to live our lives in a sacred way.

The World of the Shaman

While witchcraft is a mostly female practice, shamanism tends to be male, stemming from the hunting communities of Siberia. The word "shaman" is believed to be derived from the Tunguso-Manchurian word saman, to know. A shaman is "one who knows" and the concept of these spiritually powerful individuals extends across many cultures, including indigenous peoples of Canada, North, South, and Central America, South and East Asia, and parts of Africa. Shamanism is said to be the world's oldest religion and medical practice, its roots going back 50,000 years, as well as a spiritual discipline involving altered states of consciousness induced by the use of hallucinogenic or psychotropic plants.

Shamanism is animistic, its exponents believing that all things — animate or inanimate — are invested with spirit or consciousness. A shaman will therefore use spirit helpers from the natural world to combat hostile counterparts whose anger, jealousy, or hatred displayed toward a human causes them to attack or devour their victim's soul, resulting in sickness or death. Shamans use plants to induce a trance in order for them to give a correct diagnosis or take appropriate action. When ingested, the shaman is said to absorb the spiritual properties of these plants, allowing him to see the reality of the situation as opposed to the human world of illusions. The term "medicine man" means someone who is using the knowledge and power of life force energy.

Becoming a shaman is less a matter of personal choice than having the required predisposition and being "chosen" by the spirits. Shamanism seems to attract sensitive individuals, perhaps even those we might consider mentally ill, who can "see" spirits and therefore communicate with them. The initiation involves a form of death, in which the shaman is believed to be dismembered and returned as a new personality. This is more likely to be the result of a violent hallucinogenic experience than an actual event. There are parallels with schizophrenia, except that what is normally a private experience is shared and of benefit to the community.

Anthropologist Michael Harner, in his Foundation for Shamanic Studies in California, has pioneered a shamanic renaissance by combining authentic shamanic practice with drug-free methods of relaxation that offer people renewed focus and purpose for their lives. Harner claims that classic shamanic methods offer life-changing experiences in just a few hours, which might otherwise take years of silent meditation, prayer, or chanting.

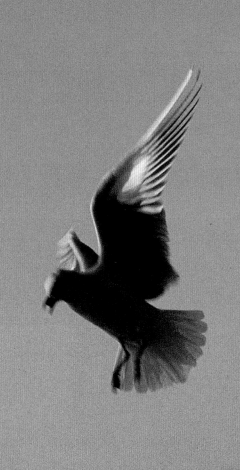

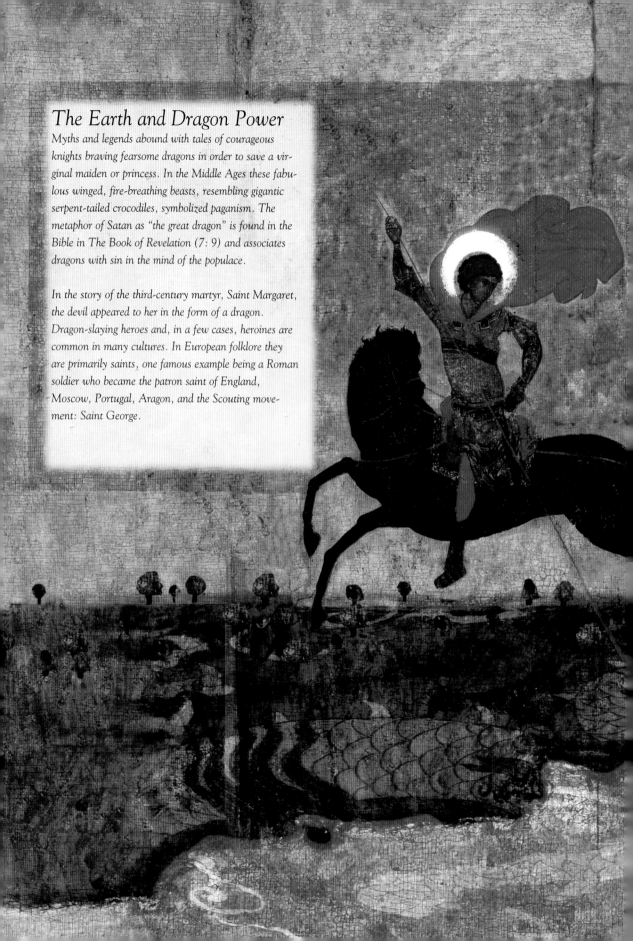

The Earth and Dragon Power

Myths and legends abound with tales of courageous knights braving fearsome dragons in order to save a virginal maiden or princess. In the Middle Ages these fabulous winged, fire-breathing beasts, resembling gigantic serpent-tailed crocodiles, symbolized paganism. The metaphor of Satan as "the great dragon" is found in the Bible in The Book of Revelation (7: 9) and associates dragons with sin in the mind of the populace.

In the story of the third-century martyr, Saint Margaret, the devil appeared to her in the form of a dragon. Dragon-slaying heroes and, in a few cases, heroines are common in many cultures. In European folklore they are primarily saints, one famous example being a Roman soldier who became the patron saint of England, Moscow, Portugal, Aragon, and the Scouting movement: Saint George.

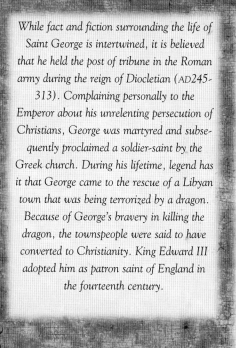

While fact and fiction surrounding the life of Saint George is intertwined, it is believed that he held the post of tribune in the Roman army during the reign of Diocletian (AD245-313). Complaining personally to the Emperor about his unrelenting persecution of Christians, George was martyred and subsequently proclaimed a soldier-saint by the Greek church. During his lifetime, legend has it that George came to the rescue of a Libyan town that was being terrorized by a dragon. Because of George's bravery in killing the dragon, the townspeople were said to have converted to Christianity. King Edward III adopted him as patron saint of England in the fourteenth century.

The legend of Saint George is an allegorical tale of the triumph of the Christian church over paganism and "forces of darkness". Pagan belief included an understanding of the primal power channelled through the earth in ley lines. Apart from their connection with sin and Satan, dragons symbolize this electromagnetic energy, or Earth chi. While the representation by dragons is not universal, the concept of subterranean energy channels crosses all cultures. In Ireland they are "fairy paths", in Polynesia "lines of light", and Australian aborigines know them as "dream paths". In the West, fuelled by the Church's distrust and fear of pagan beliefs and its desire to crush the largely maternalistic practices of wiccans, "dragon paths" were deemed to represent something negative and fearful. However, in the East, dragons are the sacred emblem of Chinese emperors and "dragon lines" highlight auspicious locations.

In the late 1970s a group of British physicists, dowsers, a chemist, an archaeologist, psychics, electrical engineers, psychologists, and "earth mysteries" workers began a research programme whose objective was: "To detect, by quantifiable physical and biological means, the manifestation of 'earth energy' at prehistoric sites and to relate this to the ultimate nature of earth energy and to the suspected prehistoric manipulation of this energy." They called it the "Dragon Project".

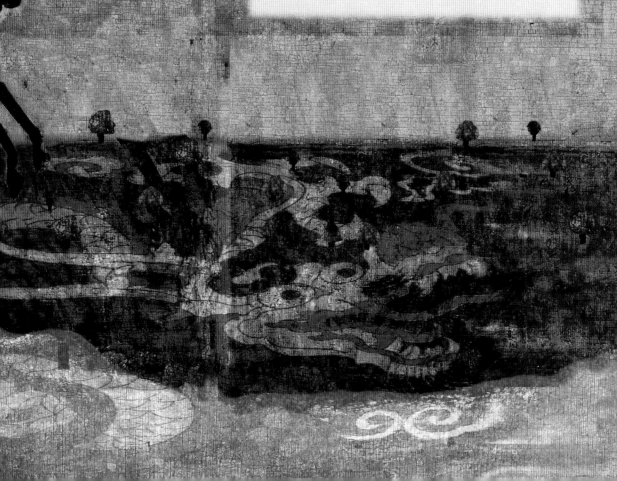

The Earth as a Creative Canvas

In the same way that, as small children, we made use of whatever came easily and cheaply to hand to create art, our ancestors utilized the Earth as both artists' materials and canvas. We are all familiar with prehistoric cave paintings, most famously the examples at Lascaux in southwestern France, those on the Tassili plateau of Algeria, and in Altamira in northern Spain. However, there are many other different illustrations of humankind's creativity and artistic endeavours, three of which are detailed below.

Scores of circular stone structures, or "medicine wheels", can be found throughout the plains and prairies of the United States and Canada. Built by Native Americans since prehistoric times and often shaped in the manner of turtles and snakes, these boulder structures are steeped in mystery. No one knows exactly why they were built, except that their astronomical alignments suggest that they were the meeting places for sacred rituals at significant times of the year. For example, the centre of the Big Horn medicine wheel in Wyoming, which has 28 lines of stones radiating as spokes, is aligned with the position of the Sun at dawn on the summer solstice. However, because the circle is symbolic of life itself, it has the potential to allow people to see reality in a different light. Hence a group of people sitting around a medicine wheel might gain a greater understanding of various perspectives, or truths, whether individually, tribally, or nationally.

Ground Sculptures

Equally mysterious are the representations of figures and animals cut into the Earth and best viewed from a distance, sometimes only by air. In the UK carvings into chalk hillsides in the southern part of England include the Long Man of Wilmington, the Cerne Abbas Giant, and the White Horse at Uffington. However, over 60 lesser-known carvings, or "terrestrial zodiacs", have been found around Britain, prompted by sculptor Katherine Maltwood's discovery in 1925 of the Glastonbury

Zodiac. These twelve figures, each representing an astrological sign and each lying within a 8-km (5-mile) radius of the other, are thought to have been mapped out in prehistoric times as sanctuaries, taking advantage of suggestive landscaping.

Ground images in other parts of the world are even more remarkable: the Serpent Mound in Ohio is an earthwork representing a partly coiled snake with an egg in its mouth and is over 381 metres (1,250 feet) long. Thought to be over 2,000 years old, it was carved into the clay by people from the Ancient Adena or Hopewell cultures, and is best seen from a viewing tower or the air. While serpents were frequently depicted on Native American artefacts, no one knows why this image was sculpted in this particular area.

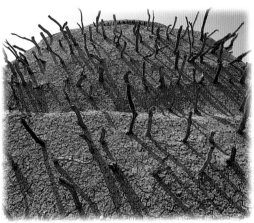

Links with extra-terrestrial beings are inevitably made with ground sculptures as immense and bizarre as those discovered cut into the Nazca desert in the foothills of the Andes. Discernible only from the air, these images of animals and other shapes are thought to have been made by the Nazca tribespeople living in the area around AD1-650. The Nazca were highly industrious and constructed aqueducts that brought water from high in the Andes mountains to the parched pampas. However, exactly how they scraped away designs hundreds of feet long that can only be appreciated from the air, without the benefit of aircraft, remains much debated, as is why they were constructed initially. However, it is clear that these "power animals" — occurring mostly in North and South American practices and beliefs — are reminiscent of labyrinths, which have long been constructed as ritual walkways for deeper self-understanding (see also pp.94-5).

Rituals featuring ground sculptures are also common throughout parts of Australia's Northern Territory, where the Gidjingali people bury their dead in the stomach of a 10.5-metre-long (33 feet) being called Ngarapia, which they draw into the sand.

The classic labyrinth design comprises pathways that travel from right to left, or left to right, analogous to the importance of both the left and right brain for creative thinking. These are unicursal paths which can, whether meditated on or physically walked around, assist in travelling deep into the subconscious. Today labyrinths are used as tools for enhancing intuition in creativity and self-discovery.

Labyrinths are found all over the world, featuring strongly in Hopi culture, throughout Europe, but particularly in Scandinavia. The Baltic coastlines of Finland and Sweden feature more labyrinths than anywhere else on Earth. Like other sacred places, labyrinths were positioned over power centres and their designs have been incorporated into Gothic churches such as Chartres Cathedral in France, itself the location of an earlier pagan site. Journeying through a labyrinth is a popular metaphor for an individual's spiritual development.

The Mathematics of Life

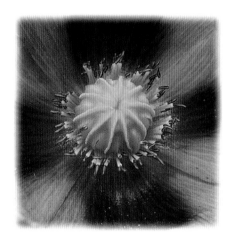

The word "geometry" means "measure of the Earth" and stems from the Ancient Egyptian practice of redefining farm boundaries temporarily covered by water during the annual flooding of the Nile. This term was thus originally coined to describe the cyclical re-establishment of the natural order of things. While quantified into the study of lines, circles, squares, and other forms, geometry was inextricably linked by the Ancient Egyptians with harmony and music, since they both conform to a common law of ratio. It is this power of ratio that gives us a sense not only of the undeniable interconnections between all things but also a more scientific understanding of how location can affect an individual.

Nature's Numbers

An appreciation of the interconnections between humankind and Nature was implicit in the design of both Ancient Greece's temples and theatres. The symmetry of form reflected universal laws that joined all forms of life, animate or inanimate. The harmony of Nature, embodied through the elementary geometric shapes of the square, triangle, or pentagon, were mirrored by the Ancients to produce an organic relationship between place and people.

Certain forms, principally the circle and the square, have long been held to have mystical and healing properties. From an esoteric perspective, squares and circles are metaphors of the universal paradox — life: it is simultaneously confining yet unlimited; manifest yet unmanifest; finite yet infinite; orderly yet chaotic; stable yet changeable and governed by cause and effect. They are, in a sense, the yin and yang of form, interlinking the rational and irrational. The importance of circles and squares for the enhancement of body, mind, and spirit lies not just in their shape but also in their proportion. This is why the medicine wheels of the native tribes of North America, such as the Big Horn medicine wheel in Wyoming (see p.58), were constructed using a measurement known as pi.

Douglas Adams, author of the *Hitch Hiker's Guide to the Galaxy*, alluded to the mathematical answer to the meaning of life when he postulated that it was the number 42. Throughout Nature self-generating patterns within plants conform to certain arithmetical sequences, including one known as the Fibonacci Series (after mathematician Leonardo Fibonacci, c.1170-1250). Always beginning with one as the first two figures, the next number in the sequence is the sum of the previous two, i.e. 1, 1, 2, 3, 5, 8, 13, 21, 34, 55, etc. What is particularly significant about the Fibonacci Series is that the two largest numbers found naturally, according to the sequence, are 144 and 233, which are in the ratio of 1: 1.1618050... If we extend the series further to the numbers 233 and 377 (144+233=377) we find they are in the ratio of 1: 1.618025... and so on, with subsequent ratios coming even closer to the figure of 1: 1.618033... the "perfect proportion", or Golden Mean.

Special Numbers

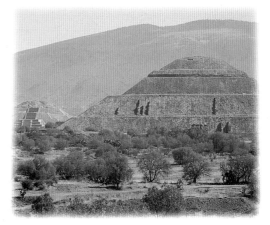

The Golden Ratio, or Mean, has been used to produce some of the world's most beautiful and awe-inspiring buildings (such as the Parthenon in Athens) and art (such as Da Vinci's *The Last Supper*). Another special number, known as pi (3.141592653...) — first calculated by Ancient Greek mathematician Archimedes (287-212BC) — is derived from the proportional relationship between the diameter of a circle and its circumference. Like the Golden Mean, pi crops up repeatedly in the natural world. The chambered nautilus shell grows according to the law known as the Golden Triangle, where the three sides are relative to 1 : pi : pi. What is significant about these and other "irrational" numbers, such as the square root of 2, and distinguishes them from other aspects of geometry, is that they do not follow any pattern. Whereas numbers like one-third (.333333...) fall into some kind of repeating sequence, this special class, like pi and the Golden Mean, are called "transcendental" and are part of a discipline known as "sacred geometry". It is interesting to note that the relaxed state of consciousness and spiritual wellbeing associated with certain ancient structures and works of art are also referred to as "transcendental". This leads one to hypothesize that sacred geometry is the universal language of the subconscious, causing the human senses, including intuition, or sixth sense, to respond so positively to the proportions, not just the aesthetics, of certain buildings such as the Taj Mahal and the pyramids of Ancient Egypt and Mexico.

Could it be that it is because modern architects have largely ignored natural laws governing pattern and form that contemporary houses and cities can be such soulless places? Ancient structures such as Stonehenge, built as a true 360° circle with rectangular stones, or the square-sided, round-cornered Pyramid of the Magicians at Uxmal, Mexico, merge both of these common geometrical forms. Such structures were built thousands of years ago and yet continue to fascinate countless visitors who travel halfway across the world to see them every year. One wonders if future generations will be similarly compelled to visit contemporary monuments, such as the UK's Millennium Dome or the US Pentagon.

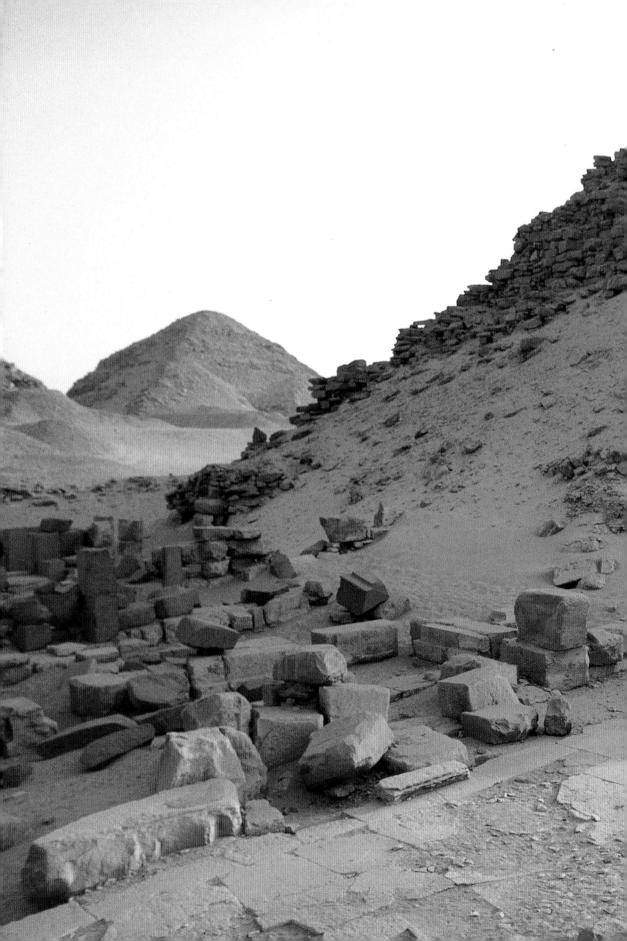

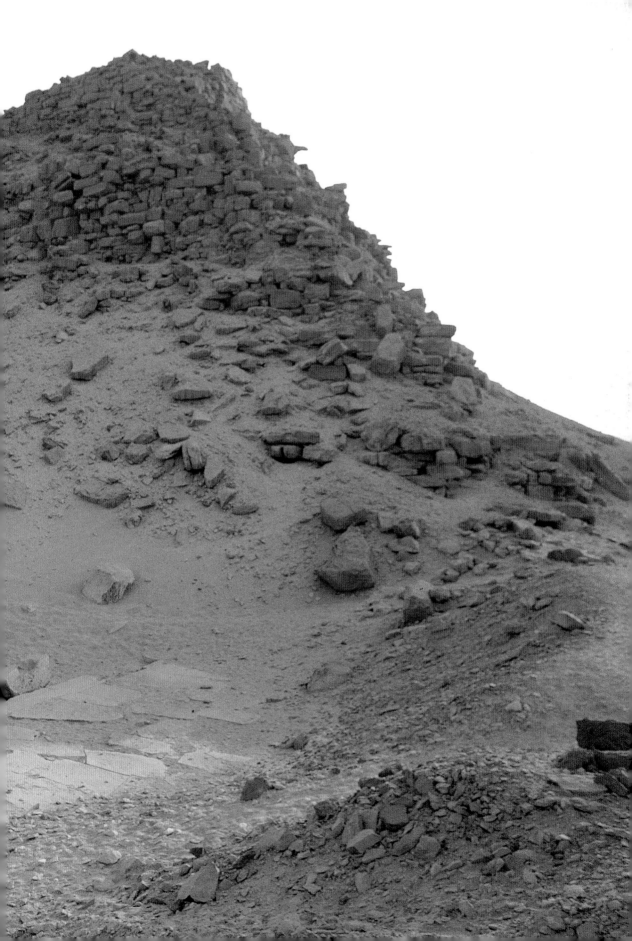

Good Vibrations

Pattern and design are inherent in Nature, from the double helix of DNA, the genetic blueprint of life, to the self-replicating lattice systems that make up natural crystals. Each of these forms is characterized by a different vibrational resonance. The Ancient Egyptians believed that sacred geometry and sound were inextricably linked. Recent research into this connection could explain one of the most puzzling phenomena of modern times: crop circles.

Ever since these mysterious patterns captured public attention in the 1970s and 1980s (although there is documented evidence of a similar phenomenon in a woodcut made in Hertfordshire, England in 1678) theorists have engaged in hot debate as to their cause. These agricultural hieroglyphics, or agriglyphs, have been discovered in the vicinity of sacred spots such as the UK's Silbury Hill, Avebury, and Stonehenge, Wiltshire, and have also materialized in fields in the USA, Canada, Australia, Scandinavia, Germany, and other parts of Europe, many over major ley lines.

One of the most spectacular agriglyphs, the Julia Set, was discovered 365 metres (1,197 feet) south of Stonehenge, Wiltshire, England, in July 1996, and, when unravelled, comprised 151 circles between 6 and 12 metres (2 and 40 feet) across and 300 metres (984 feet) long. Like the Nazca markings in Peru the dramatic scale of the geometric patterns could only be appreciated from the sky.

Crop circles have featured tens of thousands of different designs of increasing complexity, many suggestive of mandalas, stretching the claim that they are the work of hoaxers who produce them with nothing more than a few pieces of board and some ropes. Extensive laboratory analysis of the plants affected by these hitherto inexplicable patterns has revealed interesting biophysical changes, suggesting that they have been cooked from the inside or exposed to brief but intensive microwaving. Crop circle researcher, Freddy Silva, explains: "The groundwater is partly vaporized, partly sucked into the plant, thereby preventing the field from catching fire, while the stems are made supple enough to bend without cracking, enabling them to be easily manipulated into precise patterns." However, as Silva also observes, the fact that these agriglyphs conform to proportional geometry, including the Golden Mean, does not offer any helpful clues as to why they were made, by what, or by whom.

It is thought that work carried out in the 1960s by Swiss scientist Hans Jenny may offer a further clue to the mysterious appearance of crop circles. He carried out studies, or "cymatics", that involved transmitting sound through elements such as water, oil, and sand in order to capture on film the effects of vibration on physical forms. Jenny discovered that low-frequency sound produced simple, circular shapes, while higher ones increased their complexity, leading some theorists to hypothesize that it is sound that produces the phenomenon we know as crop circles. Many reports, such as that of a farmer in the wheat belt of Victoria, Australia, in 1973, also noticed an accompanying "screaming" noise around the time that these field patterns were thought to have been made.

With all the hype surrounding suggestions that extra-terrestrial beings in sound-emitting UFOs have produced crop circles in order to communicate some hitherto undeciphered messages to humankind, it is tempting to ignore the fact that Mother Earth has her own "pulse", or vibrationary rate, which, say sensitives, is changing in frequency. This has been corroborated by NASA, who have detected a rise in the "hum" emitted into space by our planet.

As Above, so Below

When looked at from the perspective of energy and not just matter, there are remarkable similarities between human beings and planet Earth. At a more universal level any illustration of atomic matter — with electrons spinning elliptically around a central nucleus — is suggestive of the way the planets in our solar system revolve around the Sun. The entire Universe (universe being derived from the Latin *unus* meaning "one" and *versus* "to turn") comprises spirals or vortices of energy. Depending on the speed at which they vibrate, these create the world of the physical (i.e. physical energy) or the metaphysical (i.e. super energy). We are only able to see physical objects that vibrate at certain frequencies, thus what we perceive as colour has no tangible component at all, but different resonances of electromagnetic radiation.

The Earth also has a subtle energy system, or life force, channelled through the Gaian equivalent of chakras and meridians. The latter are the bodily equivalent of ley lines. Interested to find out why certain ancient, sacred sites — such as stone circles, standing stones, long barrows, and churches built on pre-Christian sites — were positioned in alignment with each other, Alfred Watkins postulated the idea of ley lines or "old straight tracks". More than pathways to get our ancestors from one place to another by the shortest route (i.e. a straight line), these lines have immense astrological, energetic, and healing significance. One major ley line across the southwest of England, for example, stretches from Land's End, taking in St. Michael's Mount, the Hurlers stone circles and Cheeswring (an unusual pile of stones on Bodmin Moor, Cornwall), Glastonbury Tor, Avebury rings, and St. Michael's church, Clifton Hampden.

However, there is much more to us than our physical selves and it is here that the parallels between Mother Earth and ourselves become increasingly apparent. For example, the human energy field or aura — that pool of electromagnetic energy surrounding each of us, long depicted in religious paintings as a halo — is synonymous with the Earth's atmosphere: both are structured like the concentric layers of an onion; both offer a level of protection from external influences. In humans, the multi-layered aura (comprising the etheric, astral, and mental "selves") links our physical body with the higher systems of the psyche. This accounts for why we can sense someone looking at us, even when they are out of sight. Part of the function of the aura is to filter out unwanted or disharmonious energy from others. It is also behind the immediate attraction we can feel to individuals we do not know — as our auric field resonates in harmony with theirs. We intuitively express this universal law of like attracting like with sayings such as, "They're on my wavelength". We become sympathetic to such people in a way that is not possible if our bioelectromagnetic fields are discordant.

When the technology has been developed to enable us to read the aura other than through sensitives and esoteric healers, it is believed that this will change the face of preventive medicine, since future disease states are detectable in the auric field before they have a physical impact. This energetic information is thought to be stored in the aura, in the same way that recordings are stored on magnetic tape.

Earth's atmosphere is also made up of various energy layers that protect us from attack from all but the largest invaders from outer space and regulate the conditions that make it possible for life on this planet to exist.

Both humans and Earth generate electromagnetic frequencies, although it is unclear how these frequencies at individual locations can affect our mental, emotional, and spiritual states. Energy governs all biochemical reactions in our physical bodies, from the electrical activity of the brain, heart, and muscles, to the minute electromagnetic frequencies emanating from every living cell. These frequencies can now be measured with equipment such as electrocardiograms (ECGs) and electroencephalograms (EEGs), though ancient systems of healing have long acknowledged a subtle energy within the human body. This has been called life force, chi, or prana and is analogous with the seismic frequency, or "hum", measured by NASA. This unique bioelectromagnetic activity in the human body operates at frequencies that, until relatively recently, have proven difficult to record as they are smaller in amplitude and higher in frequency than the physiological frequencies that current scientific devices are designed to pick up.

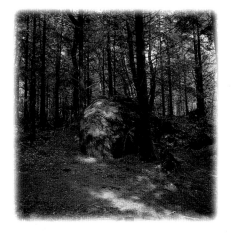

Thanks to developments with telemetry instrumentation in the UK and work by parapsychologist, scientist, and Shinto priest, Dr Hiroshi Motoyama in Japan, it is now possible to verify scientifically the existence of chi and chakras. Ancient traditions decree that life force energy is drawn into and channelled through the physical body via metaphysical vortices known as the chakras, of which there are seven principle ones (the root, sacral, solar plexus, heart, throat, third eye, and crown). While anatomically undetectable, the chakras have played a fundamental part in Eastern regimes of health and wellbeing for thousands of years and are positioned over specific, important areas of the body, such as the endocrine glands and heart. From these chakras, chi or prana flows through invisible channels called meridians. Practices such as acupuncture or shiatsu aim to unblock stagnant chi in these meridians, thus enabling energy to flow freely through the body to promote optimum health.

That many churches were built only on ley lines reflects the opposition the Catholic church felt toward long-established pagan practices. They succeeded in stamping them out, but only through compromise: legends were rewritten; symbolism was adopted; and pagan festivals and ceremonies were incorporated into the Christian calendar and reinvented. The winter solstice, or Yule, thus became Christmas, and Samhain Hallowe'en.

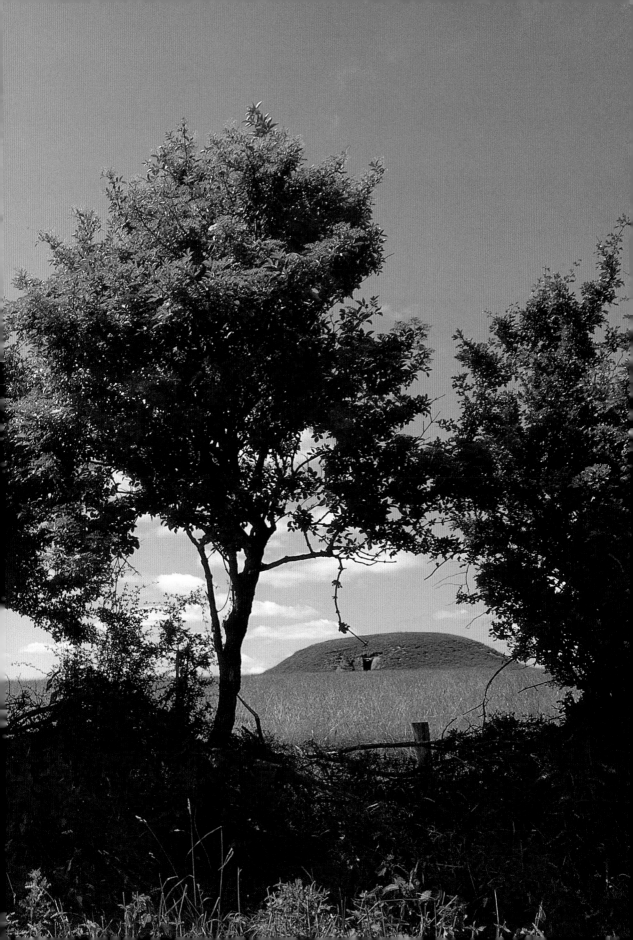

Identifying Earth Energy

The concept of ley lines is not restricted to just one culture, but is universally acknowledged. In Ireland these lines are known as "fairy paths" and in Germany as "holy lines". The Ancient Greeks referred to them as the "Sacred Roads of Hermes" — Hermes was the messenger of the gods — and the Ancient Egyptians called them the "Pathways of Min". Pacific islanders such as the Polynesians named them *te lapa*, "lines of light", while Native Americans have many names for them, including *orenda* and *manitou*. The Incas and Mayas of Mexico built their temples and pyramids on *ceque* lines and *saches* respectively, and to this day Native Australians follow the "dream paths".

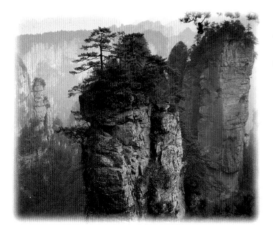

In Ancient China, where the practice of geomancy developed into a system of principles we know as *feng shui*, people believed in dragon currents, or *lung mei*, which affected the relationship between people and place. The Chinese have always been mindful of locating their temples, businesses, and homes in auspicious places — those with positive Earth chi — and are fastidious in designing architecture that blends well with the surrounding landscape. Mountains and hills that attract one kind of chi energy (see below) are deemed protectors of a city and its inhabitants, which is why Beijing, constructed and modified over centuries on geomantic principles, was located where it would be surrounded by mountains. Where such natural features did not exist, the Chinese would build them artificially, hence Coal Hill, so-called after its namesake, is now located outside the city.

Geomancers, using a variety of intuitive practices such as dowsing (see pp.86-7), would identify the invisible channels of Earth energy, or dragon currents, to ensure the harmonious positioning of buildings and tombs as well as prevent anything being erected or grown that might interfere with these subtle electromagnetic currents. The Chinese regard chi energy as representing yin and yang currents; female, yin energy flowing through low-lying areas, and male yang energy over high mountains. The most favourable positions lie where yin and yang energies intersect, hence buildings of great importance such as tombs, temples, and palaces, are often erected at these locations.

Geomancers were also astrologers — in ancient times astrology was synonymous with astronomy — and would recognize the significance of celestial alignments to these special places. It is for this reason that St. Michael's line in the UK coincides with the path of the rising sun on May Day and monuments such as Stonehenge in the UK or the pyramids in Egypt are configured according to astronomical alignments at particular times of year. That these early planners and builders commanded great knowledge across many disciplines — including arithmetic, astronomy, geometry, and sound (with regard to the resonant quality of the stones to be used) — reflects the view that buildings are more than just aesthetic attractions and are closely allied to the forms and energies of nature. They have a power that can heal the wounded spirit and fractured emotions. This multi-disciplinary, esoteric approach is, unfortunately, a far cry from the rigidly specialized activities that we engage in today and shows how far we have divorced ourselves from the rhythms of Nature.

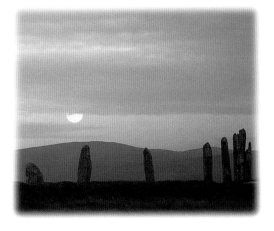

Resonant Qualities

The resonant properties of certain stones were so highly valued that prehistoric tribespeople would travel great distances to locate and bring them to designated sites, often encountering enormous transportation difficulties. The blue stones used at Stonehenge, in Wiltshire, UK, for example, are thought to have been quarried in the Preseli Mountains in South Wales, over 217 km (135 miles) away, and brought to their present site on Salisbury Plain. Why the blue stones were singled out, or indeed why different resonant stones were selected for other sites, continues to be debated. They were certainly valued for their ability to amplify sound, enabling a small group of singing or chanting adults to create the impression of a much larger gathering.

A team of scientists from Princeton University School of Engineering and Applied Science studied a number of ancient ritual sites in the UK and Ireland, including the impressive 5,500-year-old cairn at Newgrange, County Meath. They concluded that since the resonant frequencies produced within these Neolithic and Iron Age structures were within that of the adult male voice range, the design and construction of these sites were deliberately engineered to enhance human chanting.

However, some researchers have assigned the resonant qualities of design and materials with a very different role. Christopher Dunn argues in his book, *The Giza Power Plant: Technologies of Ancient Egypt*, that the Ancient Egyptians needed power tools to achieve the manufacturing precision visible in the Great Pyramid of Giza, the last of the Seven Wonders of the Ancient World. He suggests the pyramid was a power plant in itself, postulating that its constructors tapped in to the inaudible pulse, or rhythm, generated from Earth's natural mechanical, thermal, electrical, magnetic, nuclear, and chemical reactions. These resonant vibrations, coming into contact with any material that offered it the least resistance, could then be converted into airborne sound. Dunn suggests that the "thousands of tons of granite containing fifty-five percent silicon-quartz crystal" contained in the King's Chamber at Giza would then vibrate in harmony with this acoustic energy, causing what is known as the piezoelectric effect. Piezoelectricity occurs when certain crystals, particularly those of the quartz family, become stressed; this pressure causes the ions to move to opposing sides of the crystal, thereby producing different and powerful electrical charges. This phenomenon has had various commercial uses since its discovery, or re-discovery, by the Curies in 1880 and was used to produce underwater acoustic waves as an early form of submarine-detector sonar during World War I. By converting this combination of acoustic and electromagnetic energy into microwave energy through a series of complicated interactions with hydrogen, Dunn surmises that the Ancient Egyptians harnessed an ecologically beneficial power source that could power both machinery and tools — or anything else for that matter.

The science of sympathetic vibration, whereby the natural harmonizing force of the Earth is used as a source of limitless, cheap, and pollution-free power, was researched by the American scientist and inventor, John Worrell Keely, in the mid-nineteenth century. He is said to have produced a machine that could disintegrate stone, allowing certain mine owners to excavate gold that was too costly and time consuming to access by orthodox methods. On writing about this genius, the then secretary of the Theosophical Society stated: "The world will find it hard to believe that in the last quarter of the nineteenth century a man with an insight into the secret workings of nature, and a knowledge of her subtler forces... should have been left to starve, because in all the ranks of Science there was not found one man capable of understanding his colossal work..." Regrettably the same is true of today and his work remains unappreciated.

The Crystal Grid

If ley lines or energy pathways represent the meridians of Earth, then where are the planetary equivalents of the chakras, the power centres into which universal energy is channelled through all living organisms? Plato (427-347BC), imagining what the Earth might look like from space, described it as a ball made up of twelve pieces of cloth sewn together. He defined what are known as the Platonic Solids, five, three-dimensional, geometric shapes occurring in crystals, which, when meditated on, were believed to hold the key to understanding the nature of the Universe.

Research into worldwide geographical patterns implies that when Pangaea broke apart 220 million years ago (see p.26) it did so along stress lines suggestive of the first Platonic Solid, the tetrahedron. Successive fissions, leading to the formation of what we know as continental masses, occurred along lines evoking the second and third Platonic Solids, the cube and octahedron.

Russian experts writing in 1973 announced their discovery of geometric patterns of electromagnetic energy subdividing the Earth's surface into the final two Platonic Solids, the icosahedron (20 triangles) and dodecahedron (12 pentagons). Areas where the lines of these lattice-forming grids met were found to relate to phenomena ranging from the Bermuda Triangle and, lying off Japan, the Devil's Sea, to areas of high and low barometric pressure, seismic activity, major concentrations of fossil fuels, migratory routes, and the birthplaces of major cultural centres in Ancient times. These nodal vortices — centres where the electromagnetic force of the Earth is at its highest concentration — could well be the planetary equivalent of the chakras, which would provide further evidence of how energetic patterns are repeated throughout Nature, both in the human body and on Mother Earth. In the same way that balanced chakras ensure our physical, mental, emotional, and spiritual health and wellbeing, these sacred spots are vital regulators of the spiritual connection between Earth and its inhabitants.

The nodes created where grid-lines cross also coincide with over 3,000 ancient monuments and sacred places, from the Great Pyramid in Egypt to the stone head statues on Easter Island. Interestingly, the metamorphosis of this planetary crystal grid was divined by the Hopis: they spoke of the Earth's surface as resembling that of a spotted fawn whose spots move, changing the overall configuration.

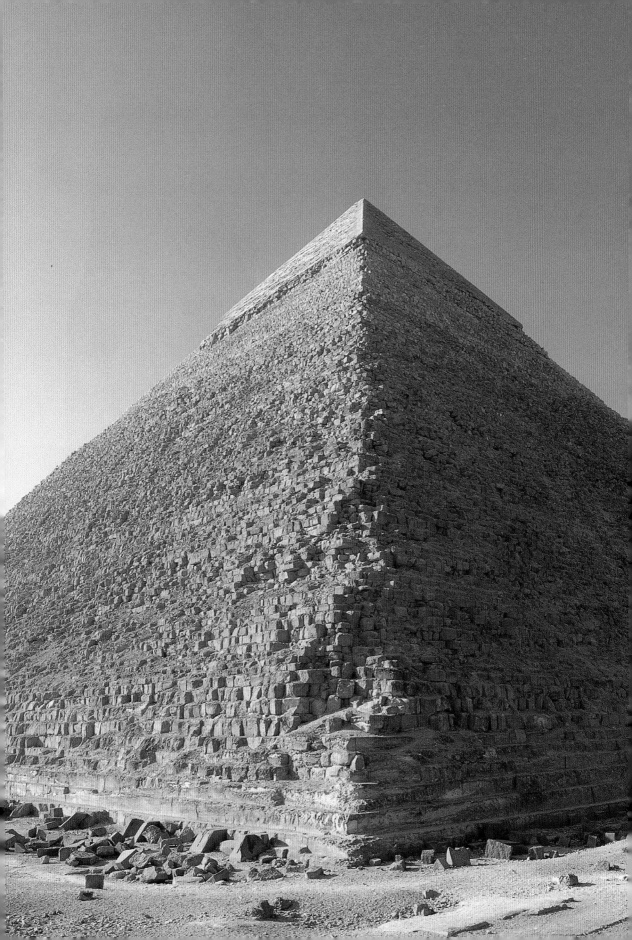

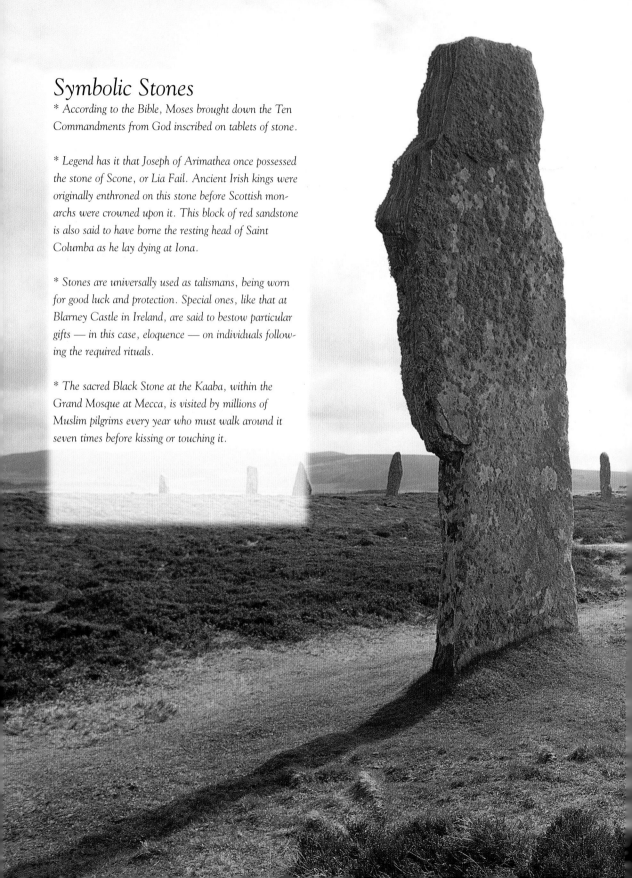

Symbolic Stones

* According to the Bible, Moses brought down the Ten
Commandments from God inscribed on tablets of stone.

* Legend has it that Joseph of Arimathea once possessed
the stone of Scone, or Lia Fail. Ancient Irish kings were
originally enthroned on this stone before Scottish mon-
archs were crowned upon it. This block of red sandstone
is also said to have borne the resting head of Saint
Columba as he lay dying at Iona.

* Stones are universally used as talismans, being worn
for good luck and protection. Special ones, like that at
Blarney Castle in Ireland, are said to bestow particular
gifts — in this case, eloquence — on individuals following the required rituals.

* The sacred Black Stone at the Kaaba, within the
Grand Mosque at Mecca, is visited by millions of
Muslim pilgrims every year who must walk around it
seven times before kissing or touching it.

No one knows exactly why stones, often transported hundreds of miles from their original resting places, were erected at certain significant sites by prehistoric humans (see also p.72). Known as megaliths, or menhirs (a Breton word meaning "long stones"), these dramatic upright blocks have been found in circular arrangements and alignments mainly in northwest Europe.

One of the most famous examples, Stonehenge, in Wiltshire, England, is said to have astronomical significance, while others, such as those found at Carnac, in France, and Avebury, southwest England, or the less conventional stone heads of Easter Island, are thought to be the planetary equivalents of acupuncture needles. In the same way that the human body has a network of subtle energy channels, known as meridians, into which acupuncturists insert their needles, megalithic standing stones are believed to have been set into the ground along ley lines to assist the free flow of Earth energies.

Because their siting was believed to have special significance, many pagan rituals concerning healing and fertility take place near these mysterious stone monuments.

* Many prehistoric stone sites are reputed to have healing powers. Legend has it that the unusual circular-holed stone at Men-an-tol, Cornwall, in England, could cure children suffering from various diseases, such as rickets, if they climbed through the hole and were then dragged around the stone three times in an anti-clockwise direction. Theorists have postulated that such sites were either positioned over areas where some form of positive Earth energy or radiation beneficial to the human organism emerged naturally, or that the stones themselves drew up this energy and amplified it for healing purposes.

* The symbolic appreciation of Gaia as possessing a body that works much like our own explains why an egg-shaped stone, regarded by the Ancient Greeks as being the most sacred in the world and part of the oracle at Delphi, was called the omphalos, or navel. This stone was believed to signify the centre of the world.

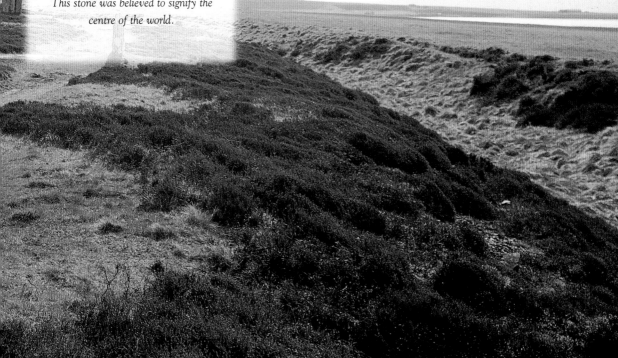

Speaking to Our Souls

We have seen, in this chapter, the extent to which pattern and rhythm are a fundamental part of Nature and that sacred architecture conforms to this natural template. The mystical significance of ancient monuments, theatres, stone circles, indeed all sacred places on this planet, lies in their ability to evoke deep feelings within us that seem to go far beyond an intellectual, aesthetic appreciation. Indeed, they seem to stir our very souls. Anyone who has visited the Blue Mosque in Istanbul, or has gazed at the north rose window of Chartres Cathedral in France. Anyone standing outside the Temple of Inscriptions at Palenque, Mexico, at Machu Picchu in Peru, or who has experienced the wonder of the pyramids, will understand that some man-made structures are more moving than others. In the same way that certain natural places, such as Mount Fuji or Niagara Falls, allow us to shed the physical pollution, emotional turmoil, and spiritual bankruptcy we all carry around, such power centres help us to regain emotional equilibrium. Nonetheless, it is important to remember that the land is not rendered sacred by structures built upon it, but that the structures are there to tap in to the sacred energy of that place.

Many of us have experienced the positive influence of certain sounds, from whale song to music. These sounds and harmonies have been found to synchronize bodily rhythms and are said to affect the chakras. However, the majority of resonances from the Earth are beyond detection by the human ear, though not by our souls. Could it be that the natural vibrational energy transferred through the thousands of sacred structures around the globe can only be sensed by the soul as they oscillate in harmony with that part of us? It is such places that imitate universal laws of pattern and proportion and by resonating with our souls, they have inspired numerous human practices from pilgrimages and vision quests to working with the beneficial vibrations of Nature and against the negative effects of geopathic stress. How we can work with these vibrations and reverse the effects of unharmonious living is the subject of Chapter Three.

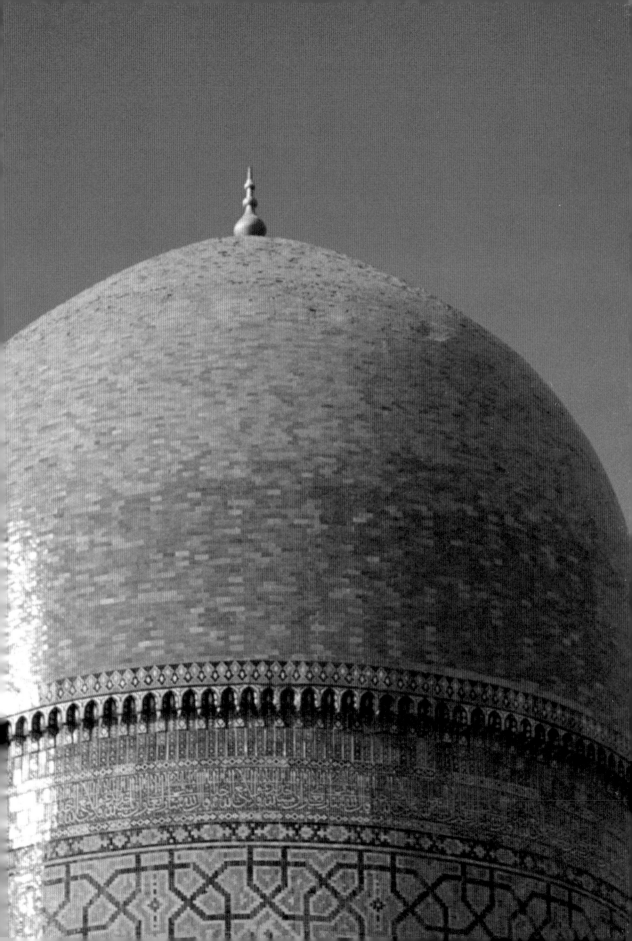

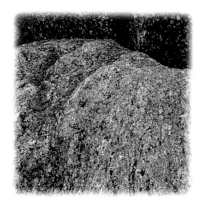

Ancient Practices

The journey to your sacred space on Earth is both an inner and an outer one. This chapter focuses on how age-old practices such as geomancy, dowsing, pilgrimage, and vision quests can assist on both of these journeys and enable us to transcend the physical, mental, emotional, and spiritual diminishment that we often experience with today's fast-paced lifestyles and high expectations. In Chapter Two we discussed how the interplay between Nature and ourselves is based on resonance — the energetic sympathy between humankind and certain special-frequency spots, often referred to as sacred places — and now we will explore the activities that ancient cultures practised across the globe to enhance and heighten life experiences. Chapter Four will investigate how you can do this, but first we will look at how these practices developed and what they involved. If we can fully understand the duality of our spiritual and physical selves, then we can contribute positively to the paradigm shift currently taking place on Earth, where as James Jeans stated fifty years ago, "... the universe begins to look more like a great thought than like a great machine". By changing our attitudes toward the world, as a precursor to changing behaviours within it, we can contribute to affecting our shared reality of Earth. All it requires is a greater emphasis on acknowledging, appreciating, and enhancing our interactive relationship with this planet.

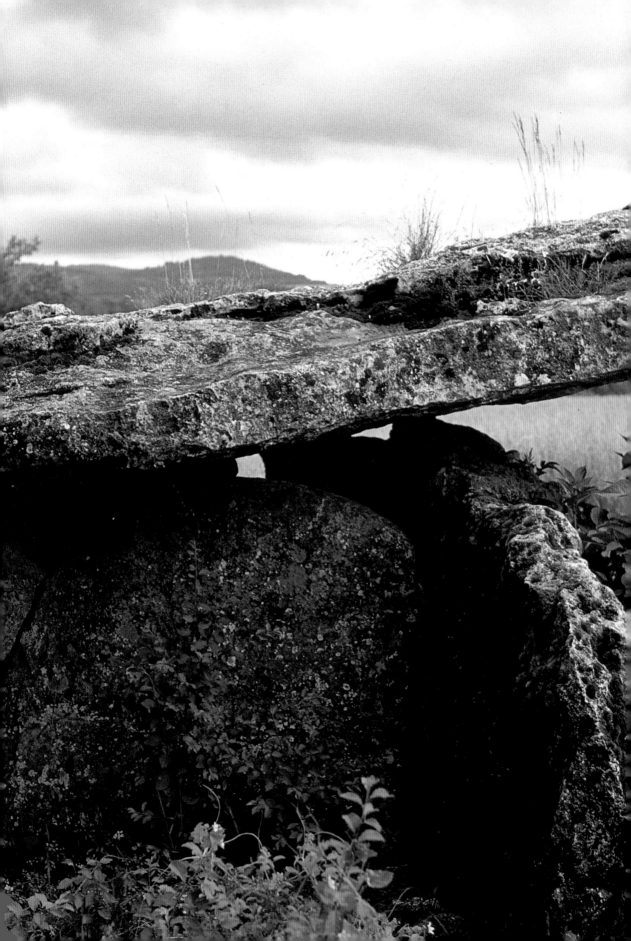

Discovering Geomantic Traditions

The Greek naturalist and writer, Pliny the Elder (AD23-79), is credited with coining the term geomancy from the Greek words *gi*, meaning "earth", and *manteia*, meaning "prophecy", although the practice itself existed many centuries before. Geomancy has been a fundamental principle of life ever since early peoples chose to site their homes, tombs, and temples at certain places rather than at others. Originally geomancy involved throwing earth or stones into the air, allowing them to fall on flat ground and then divining the relationship between the natural surroundings and humans from the patterns they made. However, the practice of divining the spirit of Earth is more wide-ranging, encompassing — at least, as it used to — sacred geometry, sound, astrology/astronomy, cosmology, architecture, dowsing, Earth acupuncture, and geology.

Nowadays we are more likely to have an appreciation of geomancy from a glossy magazine or practitioner of feng shui (see also p.112). However, no matter how the form itself has changed the principle remains the same: through studying and working in harmony with the spirit of place — a natural science in the broadest meaning of that term — people since Neolithic times have enhanced their bodies and minds, with a resulting sense of belonging, arguably the most basic, universal human need there is. While an elaborate set of practices has been built up around traditions such as feng shui and its Hindu equivalent vastu vidya (literally "dwelling science"), the most important tool that humankind has for tuning in to the power of place is our intuition, or sixth sense. For example, Native Americans chose the location for their teepees and lodges based on how they felt about a place. This makes absolute sense when you consider that individual energies are calibrated in a way that is unique to each person, so that something that suits one may not be right for another. This geomantic art of harmonious placement, therefore, does not just relate to things but more importantly, perhaps, also to people. Knowing when a place, particularly a future home, feels right for you is an important instinct to cultivate, and

Sarah wanted to move from a cramped flat to a house, but had fixed ideas about what she was looking for: the most important being to live close to the town centre. Her search, however, proved fruitless. Just as she was despairing, the agent asked if she had considered a nearby village. As she drove further into the country, she felt that she was wasting her time, yet the minute she stepped inside the house, she fell in love with it. It sits in an apple orchard, where she relishes the peace, solitude, and changing beauty of natural surroundings. Despite being remote she has never once felt vulnerable. Because she can work so much more effectively and creatively in this environment her work has taken off. She believes that this particular house was waiting for her and, although she could have paid for a feng shui practitioner to check the energies for her, nothing would have been as important, or as effective, as the sense of connection she personally feels with this place: this is where she is meant to be.

allowing "gut" feelings to influence, and sometimes even override, the often compelling focus on logic can be crucial to personal wellbeing (see facing page).

It is here that your intention (see p.86) is important. If your intention is to find somewhere to live, where you can be happy working, playing, and spending time, then this is what you need to tap in to. Geomancy is founded on the principle of intention, knowing what it is that you want to achieve. Is the intention of modern architects and builders simply to pack as many living spaces into as small an area as possible? Or is it to construct homes that can enhance their inhabitants' lives and, through that, leave them more open to the concept of community? As a home dweller, is your intention just to be closer to amenities, to find somewhere — anywhere — as long as it falls within your budget? Or is it to live in a place where your heart sings and you feel glad to be alive? Interestingly, it is usually women — often more in tune with their intuition than men seem to be — who sense when a house feels right, though they find it difficult to articulate why in a way their rationalizing partners can relate to.

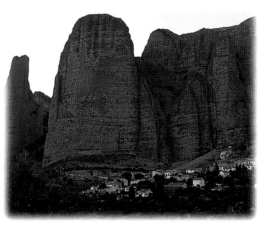

Only by switching off your conscious brain and really listening to your inner self will you stop living on this planet in a superficial and, ultimately, dehumanizing way. This involves taking time to consider, individually and collectively, what really matters to you. You may then find that where you live fails to support your life priorities in a way that it could, particularly once you absorb the notion that where you choose involves more than just putting a roof over your head.

"The land isn't sacred because the temple is here; the temple is here because the land is sacred."
A Hawaiian kahuna

Because they were so much closer to the land, embracing the magic and mystery of life as a matter of course, our ancestors naturally sought to locate themselves where the Earth energies were most congruent with their own. We too can do this if we open our minds to believing that the power of place relies less on the physical and more on the psychical.

Negative Earth Energies

The importance of beneficial Earth energies is perhaps better understood when we consider what can happen when we are exposed to its harmful energies. According to the principles of yin and yang, every positive force is countered by a negative. Just as certain frequencies can be beneficial, both physically and mentally, to human beings — which accounts for why we flock to places that make us feel good — so are some Earth energies linked with serious human illnesses such as cancers, multiple sclerosis, myalgic encephalomyelitis (ME), and migraines.

Geopathic stress is the name given to naturally occurring Earth radiation that becomes distorted by underground water, certain mineral concentrations, and the positioning of deeply anchored man-made structures, and has implications for the healthy functioning of our immune system. Ancient cultures across the globe recognized that there are places with dangerous electromagnetic energies, where it would be ill-advised to live or work because of the likelihood of suffering from a subsequent geopathogenic sickness. Prompted by scientific investigations into the ancient practice of water divining, or dowsing (see p.86), geopathic stress is now beginning to be taken seriously again.

Precisely why underground water should have such a deleterious effect remains debatable. One German hydraulics engineer has postulated that nuclear reactions taking place constantly at the Earth's core produce neutron radiations. When exposed to the friction produced by subterranean streams these can modify and concentrate into a lethal, noxious mixture. These energies then seep up through the earth and in turn disrupt the delicate homeostasis of living creatures above.

While scientists study and accept the magnetic sensitivity of animals and birds, it may still be a long time before the orthodox community fully acknowledges our own vulnerability to the Earth's magnetic field, both internally and externally, positively and negatively.

Old wives' tales warn against sleeping in a place where a cat or dog refuses to lie down. Similarly, Irish farmers sensitive to the behaviour of their livestock near traditional "fairy paths" avoid penning or herding animals over dysfunctional geopathic zones. However, if you have neither a large pet nor the inclination to herd animals through your living and sleeping areas, you may wish to take precautions to identify the extent of geopathic stress in your home or workplace.

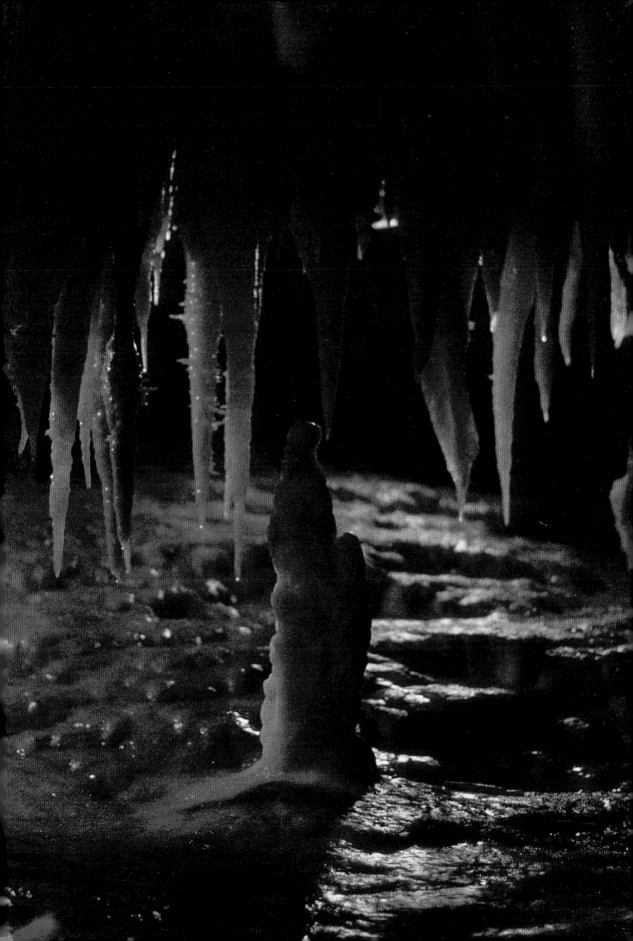

Tapping in to the Earth's Energies

How to make dowsing rods

* Take two wire coat hangers and two plastic ballpoint pens, with insides removed.

* With wire cutters, snip each hanger halfway along one short side, and then at the further end of the long side, just before it bends back on itself.

* Straighten the bend to form a right angle and place the shorter length in each of the plastic sleeves.

* When you hold the rods in your closed palms they should swivel freely.

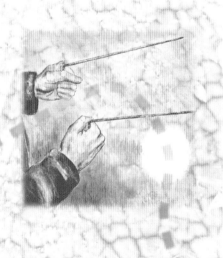

Dowsing is an age-old tradition, popularly thought of as water divination, for those with special powers. However, we all have the in-built capacity to detect energetic variations in our environment, in the same way that we experience "gut" feelings. Unfortunately in today's rationally minded society, where logic prevails, we have largely divorced ourselves from the vibrational qualities of Nature and need to re-educate ourselves in such ancient arts.

Dowsing can be undertaken by anyone with the will to do it and is used to survey sacred and other sites, to prospect for minerals and water, to trace lost objects (or even missing persons), to highlight areas of geopathic stress, and also to locate dis-ease. Devices used vary from forked branches, pendulums, or a pair of angle rods. These simply help dowsers focus and read their innate psychic awareness of electromagnetic energy. The result depends on your intention (see p.83).

Successful dowsing depends on the clarity of your intention and, paradoxically, detaching yourself from the need to achieve a particular result. It is therefore counterproductive to "try" too hard. Because it involves tapping in to your innate sensitivity and Higher Self, it is essential to dowse only when you are physically well, emotionally balanced, and mentally open.

Focus on your intention. Then start to walk slowly but purposefully around the area, holding your rods and being sensitive to their movements. You could also try asking for the support of your devas (see pp.130-1). Whatever area your rods help you to locate, be guided by your intuition. Does the site feel right? Is this a place to make you feel motivated? In the final analysis, your sacred spot should be where you want it to be. Always be aware that your rods will be sensitive to water pipes and electric cables, which can influence the result, particularly when you are new to dowsing or when your mind wanders.

• Path taken during dowsing

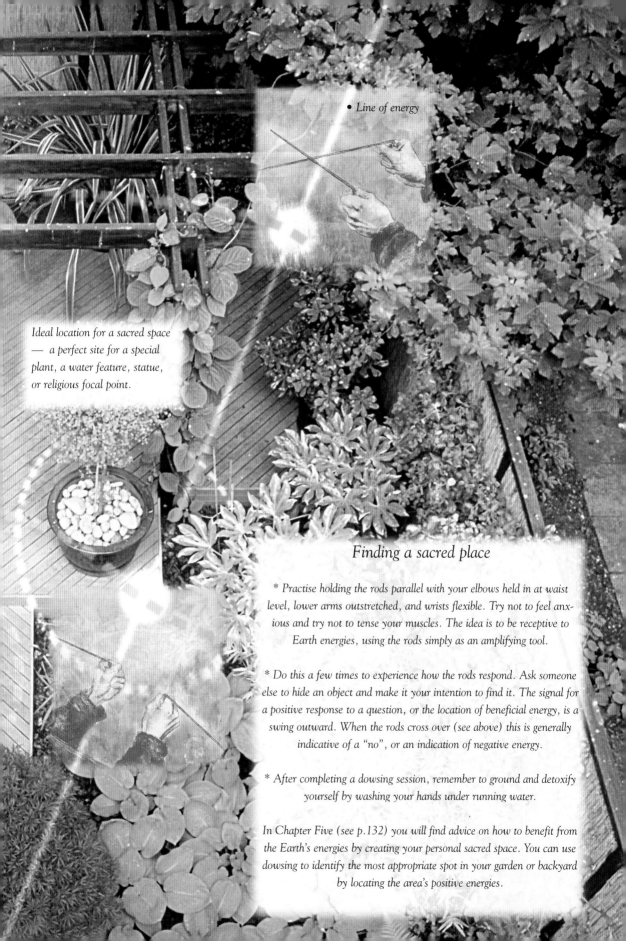

• Line of energy

Ideal location for a sacred space
— a perfect site for a special
plant, a water feature, statue,
or religious focal point.

Finding a sacred place

* Practise holding the rods parallel with your elbows held in at waist
level, lower arms outstretched, and wrists flexible. Try not to feel anx-
ious and try not to tense your muscles. The idea is to be receptive to
Earth energies, using the rods simply as an amplifying tool.

* Do this a few times to experience how the rods respond. Ask someone
else to hide an object and make it your intention to find it. The signal for
a positive response to a question, or the location of beneficial energy, is a
swing outward. When the rods cross over (see above) this is generally
indicative of a "no", or an indication of negative energy.

* After completing a dowsing session, remember to ground and detoxify
yourself by washing your hands under running water.

In Chapter Five (see p.132) you will find advice on how to benefit from
the Earth's energies by creating your personal sacred space. You can use
dowsing to identify the most appropriate spot in your garden or backyard
by locating the area's positive energies.

Making a Spiritual Journey

There is something very special about making a pilgrimage, despite the fact that travelling around the globe, often to places of great beauty or spiritual significance, has never been easier to arrange. This kind of ritualistic journey is analogous to the soul's quest for enlightenment. Others may accompany you, but it is the unique mission that you have set yourself — in life, as on the pilgrimage — that is the crucial factor. A pilgrimage has the ability to change you, irrevocably, forever. It challenges you to reassess your values, your sense of self, and how you best contribute to the world. A degree of physical risk and emotional vulnerability may be involved, the pain of which can help you to re-evaluate the joy your life has to offer, rather than focusing on the negative. In so doing you change from being a sightseer —someone who looks on but does not participate — to a person who involves themselves fully in life, physically, mentally, emotionally, and spiritually.

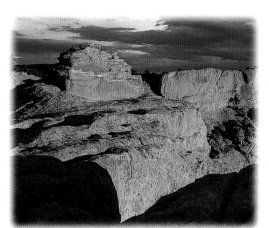

Making a Pilgrimage

No one knows exactly when the ritualistic journeying we call pilgrimage first became a valuable part of human endeavour, but the practice transcends time and culture. A pilgrimage is a reciprocal experience in as much as the individual travels to a specially designated spot in order to return to a sense of spiritual and psychological balance and regain a sense of connection and power. Sometimes, in the case of places such as Lourdes, in France, it is also to physically heal. However, pilgrimage is a time to give as well as to receive. This can mean to acknowledge and pay homage to the spirit of place by offering a physical gift or prayer, or to take part in a procession or a form of creative expression such as singing or dancing.

Pilgrimage is, paradoxically, a simultaneously individual experience and one that unites humankind. Many pilgrims report an overwhelming desire to be alone and hence actively dissociate themselves from other travellers. This desire to distance oneself from others, to abstain from superficial conversation, should not be interpreted as being directly anti-social, for the personal space it allows the person heightens their experience of oneness with their God. Any woman who has experienced the overriding need to virtually hibernate for the few days leading up to giving birth will understand how this withdrawal is an important precursor to producing new life. On a pilgrimage, the desire to withdraw socially relates to the rebirth of your Higher Self. The choice of certain remote and often quite inaccessible sites is analogous to the challenge of reaching beyond the mask of personality, or ego, to the inner diamond that is the soul, or Higher Self. It is far harder to achieve these levels of self-mastery oneself than it is to tell someone how to do it. Only by putting theory into practice, by undertaking some form of personal pilgrimage and allowing long-ignored, painful emotions to surface, can you acquire true wisdom, compassion for others, and unconditional love — or that which some call God.

As far as an experience of union is concerned, pilgrimage is common to many orthodox religions: many Christians repeatedly make their way to Lourdes; Muslims are expected to visit Mohammed's birthplace at Mecca at least once in their lifetime; millions of Hindus ritually wash themselves in the River Ganges annually; and countless Jews daily push written prayers into gaps in the Wailing Wall of Jerusalem. However, in many places of pilgrimage the emphasis is on the sacred geography, rather than on any particularly holy figure or ascribed set of beliefs. Such is the appeal of Mount Fuji in Japan, Glastonbury Tor in England, the Externsteine, or Dragon Stones, in northern Germany, and the sacred mountain of Croagh Patrick in County Mayo, Ireland. These places seem to accord the visitor an overwhelming sense of inner peace and connection to Nature, which could be described as a sense of what is often termed enlightenment.

Sacred Places

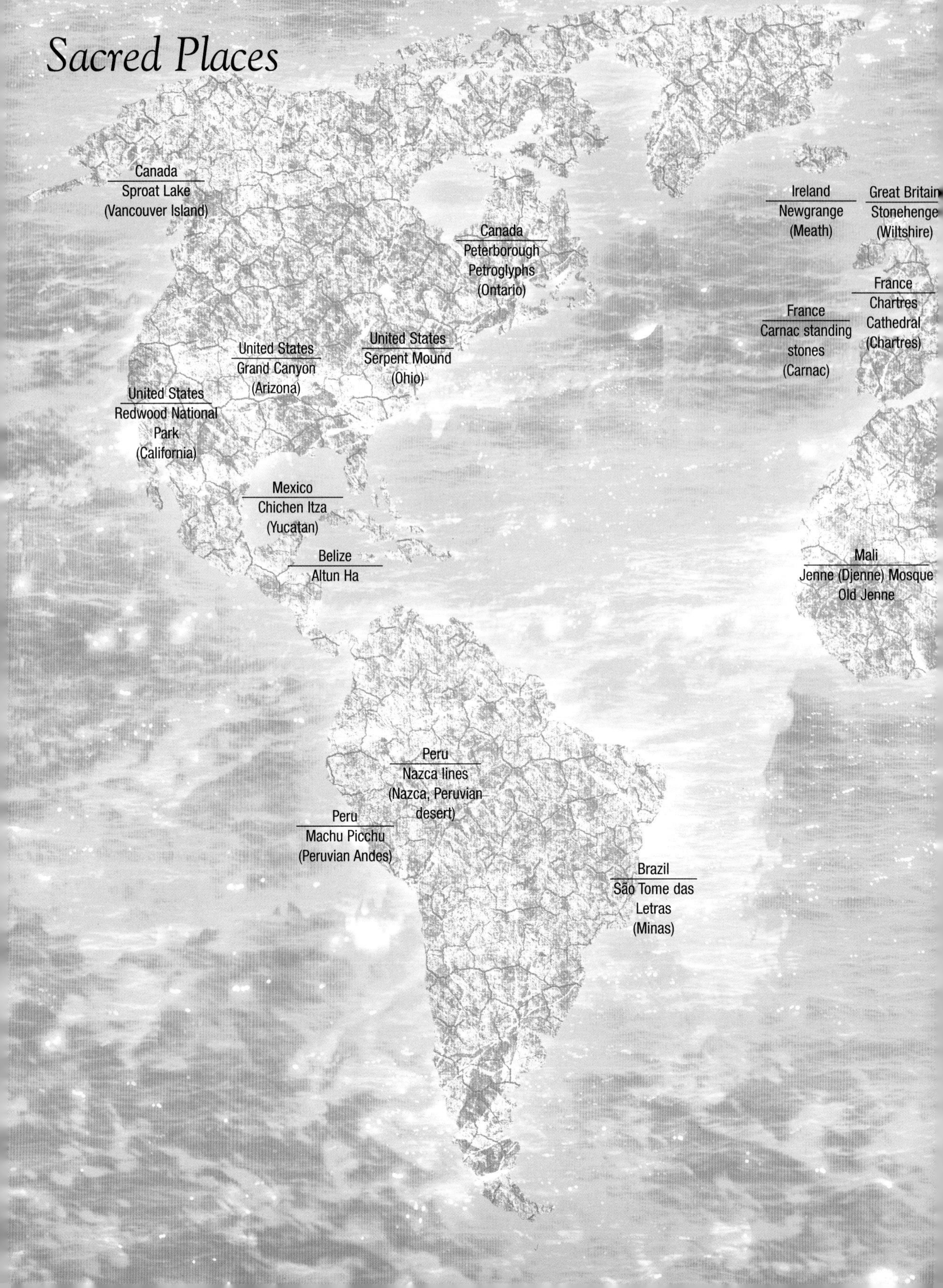

Canada
Sproat Lake
(Vancouver Island)

Canada
Peterborough
Petroglyphs
(Ontario)

Ireland
Newgrange
(Meath)

Great Britain
Stonehenge
(Wiltshire)

France
Chartres
Cathedral
(Chartres)

United States
Grand Canyon
(Arizona)

United States
Serpent Mound
(Ohio)

France
Carnac standing
stones
(Carnac)

United States
Redwood National
Park
(California)

Mexico
Chichen Itza
(Yucatan)

Belize
Altun Ha

Mali
Jenne (Djenne) Mosque
Old Jenne

Peru
Nazca lines
(Nazca, Peruvian
desert)

Peru
Machu Picchu
(Peruvian Andes)

Brazil
São Tome das
Letras
(Minas)

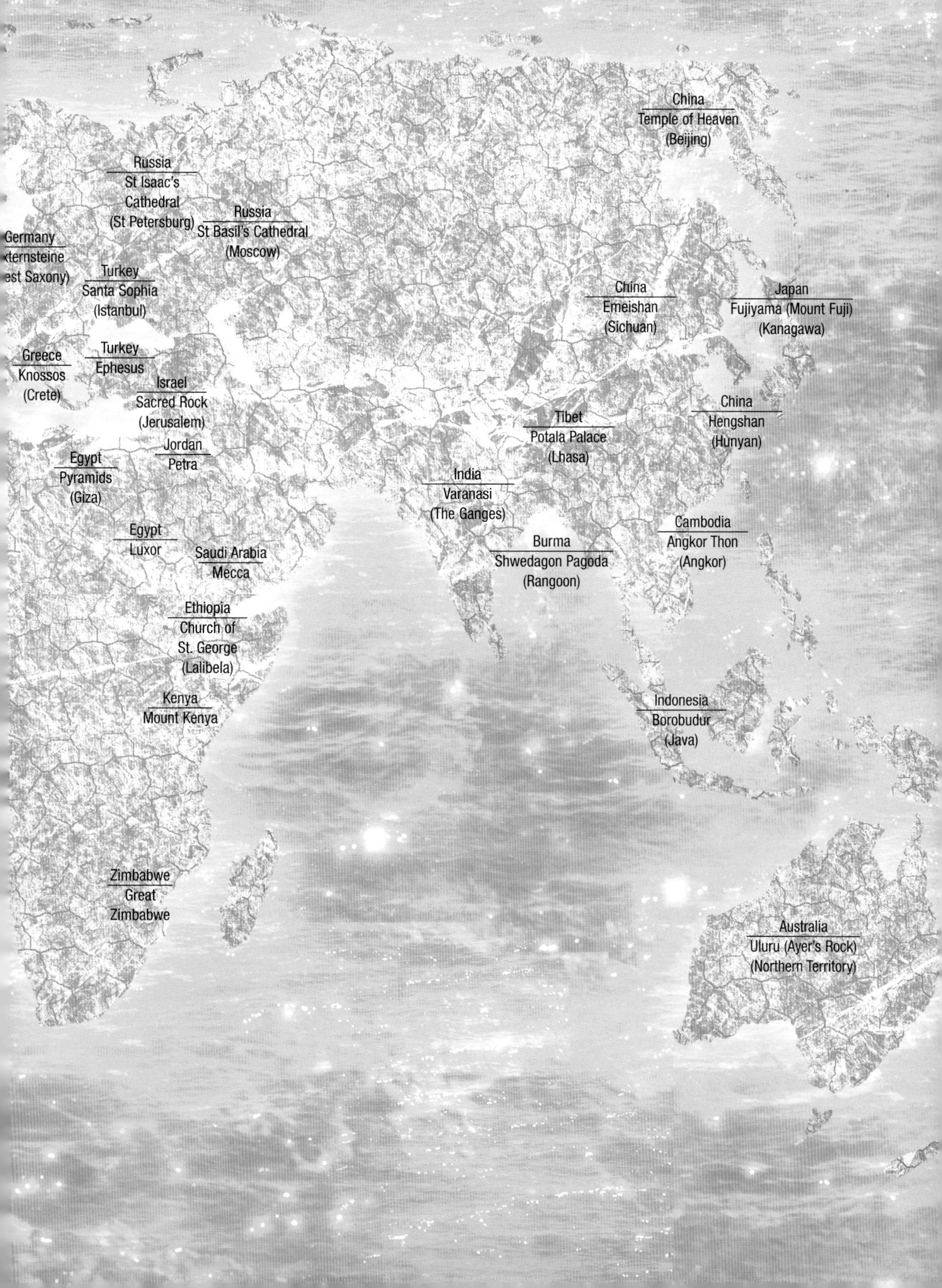

China
Temple of Heaven
(Beijing)

Russia
St Isaac's
Cathedral
(St Petersburg)

Russia
St Basil's Cathedral
(Moscow)

Germany
xternsteine
est Saxony)

Turkey
Santa Sophia
(Istanbul)

China
Emeishan
(Sichuan)

Japan
Fujiyama (Mount Fuji)
(Kanagawa)

Greece
Knossos
(Crete)

Turkey
Ephesus

Israel
Sacred Rock
(Jerusalem)

China
Hengshan
(Hunyan)

Tibet
Potala Palace
(Lhasa)

Jordan
Petra

Egypt
Pyramids
(Giza)

India
Varanasi
(The Ganges)

Cambodia
Angkor Thon
(Angkor)

Egypt
Luxor

Saudi Arabia
Mecca

Burma
Shwedagon Pagoda
(Rangoon)

Ethiopia
Church of
St. George
(Lalibela)

Indonesia
Borobudur
(Java)

Kenya
Mount Kenya

Zimbabwe
Great
Zimbabwe

Australia
Uluru (Ayer's Rock)
(Northern Territory)

Looking Within

The practice of communing in solitude with Nature is linked with certain religious or historic figures and generally precedes an important change or event in their lives. In the Bible Jesus goes into the wilderness early in his ministry, where he fasts for forty days and nights while confronting temptation by the Devil.

There is no need to travel great distances to engage in a journey of self-discovery. In some practices it is the ritual involved that affects a particular outcome, as with "vision quests". Vision quests are sometimes thought to be exclusive to Native Americans, but they also feature in many shamanic societies, where reality is considered to comprise both the material and the unmanifest and every single thing — animate or inanimate — is believed to possess a spirit.

At a designated, isolated, spot thought to be imbued with special potency and power, the seeker embarks on a period of sensory deprivation involving seclusion, fasting, prayer, and introspection. This results in what is known as a vision state, an altered state of consciousness often referred to as ecstasy. The individual experiences a psychological sense of disembodiment and may merge with his or her guardian spirit — usually an animal — in order to acquire certain characteristics and knowledge.

Hills, cliffs, caves, trees, and unusual rock formations are all considered suitable places for a vision quest. This rite of passage is not a once-in-a-lifetime event, but, as with the Comanches of North America, takes place at particular junctures throughout life, in order to reconnect the individual with the spirit world through Nature. Another form of questing, or journeying, involves using labyrinths (see p.94).

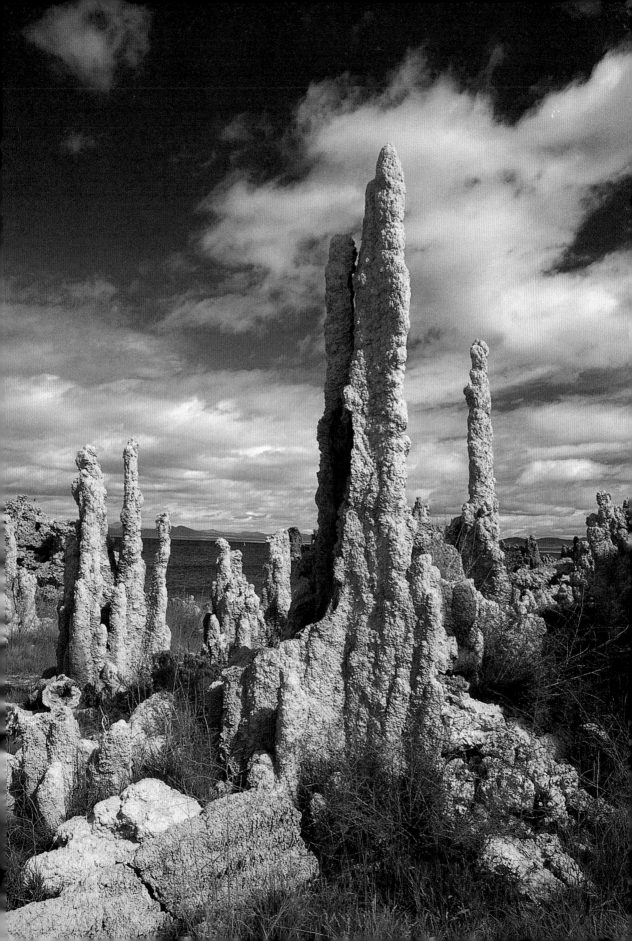

The Labyrinthine Journey

The word labyrinth is Greek in origin and is thought to be connected with *labyris*, the double-headed axe, symbol of Ancient Crete, where one of the most famous labyrinthine myths, of Theseus and the Minotaur, was set. This mythical labyrinth takes the form of a building made up of interconnected passages, so tortuously designed that it was easy to get lost and be unable to find your way out. The word labyrinth has also been used to describe the intricate, maze-like patterns found on the floors of Gothic cathedrals and churches. The connection between labyrinths and Mother Earth is epitomized by the Hopi Native American symbol, known as the Classical Seven Path Labyrinth, which is associated with the sacredness of Nature because of the spiralling disposition of plants. These sacred gateways to our inner selves are also reminiscent of what is called kundalini energy, which, in the Hindu tradition, is coiled in the form of a serpent goddess at the root chakra, and then piercing each chakra in turn as it moves up the body until it reaches the crown. When this happens, a person is said to have achieved enlightenment.

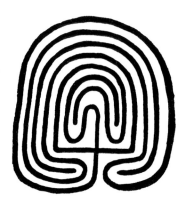

Labyrinths can be regarded as metaphors for a period within the process of self-mastery, commonly called "the dark night of the soul". In order to transcend our egos and become more in tune with our Higher Selves, there comes a time when we need to confront our inner demons — the dysfunctional beliefs, attitudes, and fears we have carried with us from childhood, perhaps even from previous lives. The story of Theseus and the Minotaur — monstrous half man, half beast, who resided in a mythical labyrinth within the Ancient Cretan capital of Knossos — is perhaps symbolic of the spiritual self prevailing over the base self, the one that connects us most with the animal kingdom. It is interesting to note that Theseus, later king of Athens, was not a god but a mortal, who nevertheless went beyond the boundaries of humankind, even venturing into and returning from Hades, the Ancient Greek underworld, home of the dead. By a process of creative thinking, that is by using a ball of yarn to help him retrace his steps out of that dark, intricate maze, Theseus was able to make his way calmly into the heart of the labyrinth and slay the Minotaur, thus putting an end to his annual sortie to devour nine male and nine female virgins.

The possible impact of this legend on medieval Europe is apparent in the semantics of the word clew, or clue: that which contributes toward solving a problem, originally meaning a ball of thread. Its popularity prompted an interest in laying out labyrinths in cathedrals, where they became a meditative tool. The link between labyrinths and pilgrimage, the latter often undertaken by people on their knees, led to many labyrinths being called Jerusalem. The existence of the most complex labyrinths, one of the most famous in Chartres Cathedral, is evidence of the long, arduous, but ultimately spiritually uplifting practice of pilgrims through the centuries.

The lesson to be drawn from labyrinths clearly mirrors many lines of spiritual teachings: we each hold the answers to our deepest psychological challenges within ourselves. We can face our most terrifying, subconscious fears — and return unscathed, as Theseus did — by engaging in simple pursuits, by taking up our courage, and by engaging our inner calm. As a metaphor for human spiritual development, meditating on the intricate pattern of a labyrinth, either by tracing one with your index finger or by walking around a full-sized one, can help you come to terms with the way you approach life. As you follow the path, reflect on the following: do you consider life to be full of insurmountable challenges, pitfalls, and dark experiences or is it rather an exciting and mysterious adventure for you? Do you accept that life's journey is full of unexpected detours or do you wish that it was a predictable straight path? Are you able to maintain a certain perspective on your life and face events with an open mind or do you fight to maintain control of your life at all times? Is life all about reaching your destination or are you fully experiencing this wonderful journey? What is your goal in life? What might the centre of the labyrinth represent for you?

The Final Journey

We may emerge from our mother's womb at birth, but it is to our Earth Mother that we return when we die. Because most humans find death so psychologically difficult, different cultures have tried to devise means of coping with and maintaining control over this unavoidable fact of life by employing special burial rites and rituals. Early cultures buried their dead in the foetal position rather than outstretched, as is usual today. This perhaps suggests a belief in returning the body to Mother Earth to be reborn. Royalty and other important people, such as those buried at Ur, Mesopotamia, 5,000 years ago, were also accompanied to the afterlife by those who had been of service to them.

For centuries, in many country areas in the UK, a dying person would be placed on the earthen floor to speed their passing, a practice linked with the biblical assertion that God formed humankind from the Earth and to the Earth we must return. The practice of burying the dead in a casket or coffin, accompanied by some of their most precious possessions, such as jewellery and clothes, and also necessary food, money, or tools, can be traced back to Palaeolithic times. This indicates a belief in immortality and that the afterlife was thought to be no different from this one. The ancient Persian religion, Zoroastrianism, decrees that, in order to avoid contaminating the Earth's holy elements, corpses should be placed on platforms on high ground, where the bodies can be eaten by vultures, or disintegrate naturally. Many cultures place great importance on the direction in

Exactly why humans — the only species to do so — bury their dead is open to speculation. However, this near-universal practice, which has become more elaborate as the centuries have gone by, and is modified only according to different cultural rituals, is thought to be concerned more with humankind's esoteric beliefs about death than with sanitation.

"In the sweat of thy face shalt thou eat bread till thou return unto the ground; for out of it wast thou taken: for dust thou art and unto dust shalt thou return."

"Therefore the Lord God sent him forth from the garden of Eden, to till the ground from whence he was taken."
Genesis 3:19, 4:23, The Bible

which a body is buried. For Muslims, the right side must face Mecca. Buddhists lie with their heads pointing north, shamans face the land of their ancestors, while Ancient Egyptians faced west in accordance with the setting of the Sun.

Freedom to be buried how and where you choose is now gaining in popularity. In response, many nature reserve burial grounds are being developed, offering an economical, eco-friendly, and spiritually appealing means of burial. These green, or woodland, sites allow individuals to be buried in a biodegradable shroud or cardboard coffin, so that they can decompose freely and feed the tree planted over them. This practice cuts down on wasteful wooden coffins, polluting cremation, and the vast tracts of land consumed by cemetaries.

Engaging in rites and ceremonies that helped the dead in their journey may have been a vital way for Stone Age peoples to accept the psychologically challenging fact of their mortality. It also highlights the acknowledgement of humankind that something of us survives our physical death — that ineffable aspect of human nature we call "the spirit" or "soul".

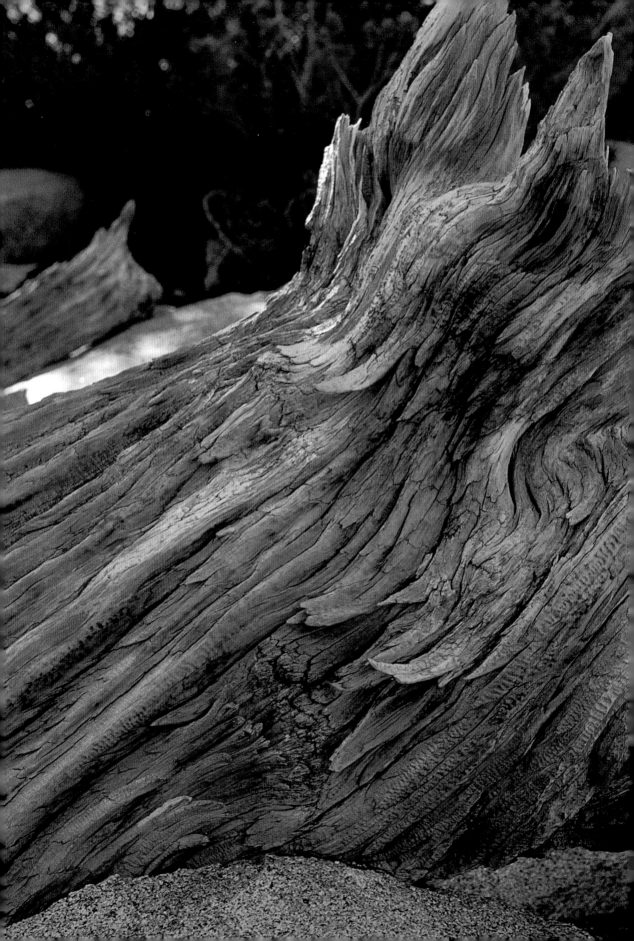

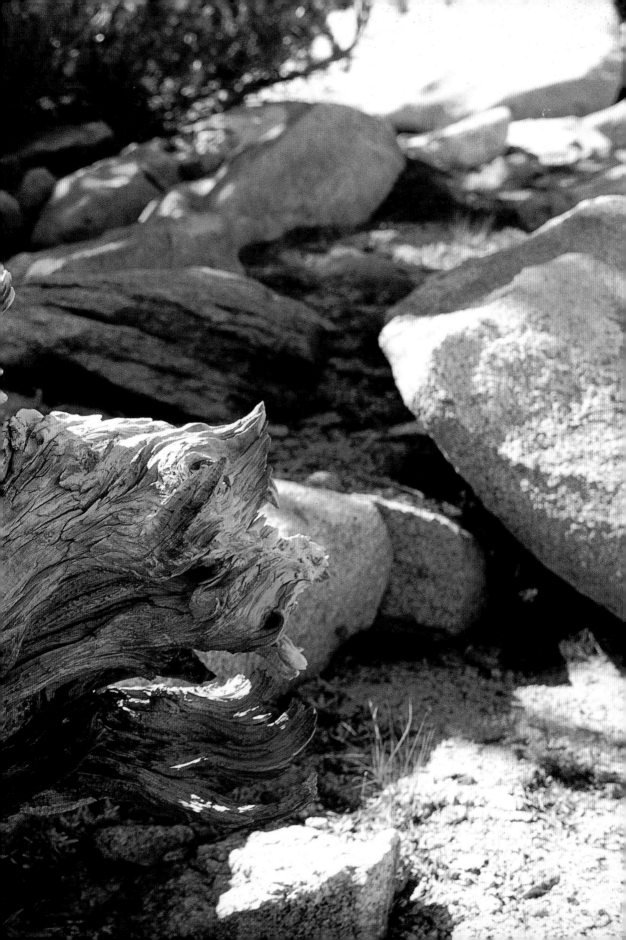

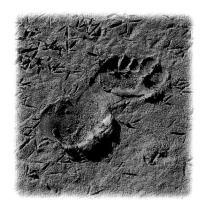

You and Your Earth

This chapter is divided into three sections: you; your indoor environment; and your outdoor environment. Within each are things you can do to align yourself with the healing energies of Earth. The key principle is balance, demonstrated perfectly by Nature, which maintains homeostasis despite challenging circumstances. The suggestions relate to life as a whole, combining to express a realistic form of spiritual practice to reconnect yourself to the Source, the Divine, or God.

We start with you. The first step in this process of personal ecology involves clearing and balancing your own energies. This preparation will help you tune in to your environment, so that you are more receptive to intuitive messages and life's signposts. Such a process has been called many things, though voluntary simplicity, the fusion of Earthly pragmatism and spiritual abundance, defines it neatly. There are several practical steps you can take to reduce the complexity of your life that will bring immediate benefits. Physically, living simply helps reduce stress levels. Psychologically, it opens you up to the energetic channels of communication — your intuition, or sixth sense, which we often find hard to tap in to because of our materialistic tendencies. Spiritually, voluntary simplicity prompts you to put your belief into practice, to "walk your talk", and demonstrate your belief in an abundant and generous Universe.

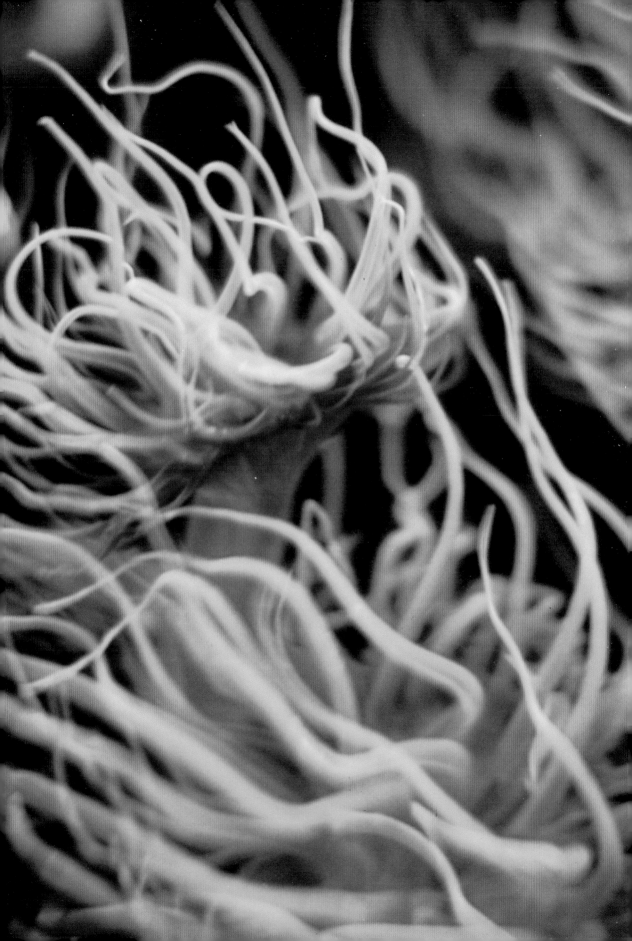

The Ten-Point Life Simplification Plan

If you feel that you are living life on a tread-mill and you want to get off, try some of the following suggestions:

1. Make a daily appointment with yourself

Take twenty minutes to shut yourself away and ask what is important to you. How could you simplify your life — let it become more meaningful and enjoyable? We tend to believe that solutions are provided by others, but we each hold the answer to every single challenge facing us, deep within our souls. To access these answers we need to remove ourselves periodically from the hubbub of everyday noise and allow the whisper of our intuition to penetrate our consciousness.

2. Cultivate simple values

Use your times of reflection to rediscover the universal laws that govern Nature and detach yourself from the need to always be doing something. Stop trying to control your life and allow it instead to unfold by itself. Do less and accomplish more. Just as Nature is cyclical and subject to the seasons, so too are events in life: whatever is going wrong in your life will change for the better in the same way that winter will always turn into spring.

3. Take a good look around your home

Clear out anything that does not hold personal meaning for you: unwanted knick-knacks, old clothes, piles of magazines. Which of your possessions are really important and which are merely constant reminders of the complexity and stagnation within your life? Re-energizing your personal space by clearing out clutter plays an important part in bringing you toward a fresh perspective on life.

4. *How frugally can you live for a month?*

Look critically at your living expenses and see where you can save. What about those duplicated insurance policies? Do you really read every newspaper and magazine you buy? Is lack of menu-planning the reason why your food bills are so high? Could you team up with others to bulk-buy regular items?

5. *Could you give more?*

Give ten per cent of your savings to a charity, religious organization, or group whose needs are greater than yours. Money is an energy that needs to flow out as well as in to your life. Gratitude for what you have and generosity toward others are two of the spiritual keys to happiness. You will soon realize that you are prosperous in ways that have nothing to do with amassing money.

6. *Manage your time*

Divide your activities into things you really need to do yourself, things you can delegate, and those that can be deferred to another time. The more you become focused and organized about your life and work, the more you will stop fire-fighting and enjoy each precious moment. With a calmer perspective, you will undoubtedly find that time is not the enemy you once thought.

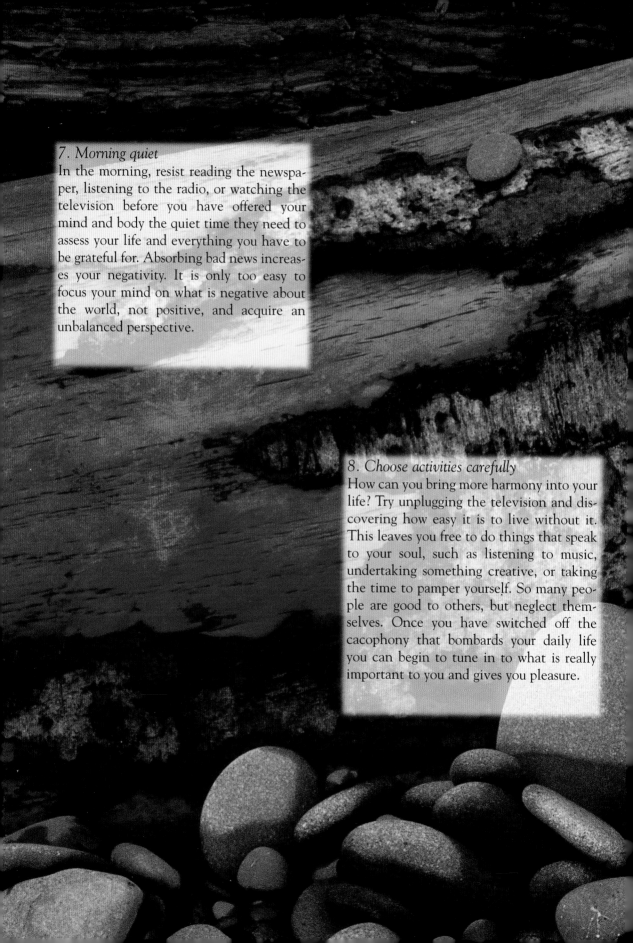

7. Morning quiet

In the morning, resist reading the newspaper, listening to the radio, or watching the television before you have offered your mind and body the quiet time they need to assess your life and everything you have to be grateful for. Absorbing bad news increases your negativity. It is only too easy to focus your mind on what is negative about the world, not positive, and acquire an unbalanced perspective.

8. Choose activities carefully

How can you bring more harmony into your life? Try unplugging the television and discovering how easy it is to live without it. This leaves you free to do things that speak to your soul, such as listening to music, undertaking something creative, or taking the time to pamper yourself. So many people are good to others, but neglect themselves. Once you have switched off the cacophony that bombards your daily life you can begin to tune in to what is really important to you and gives you pleasure.

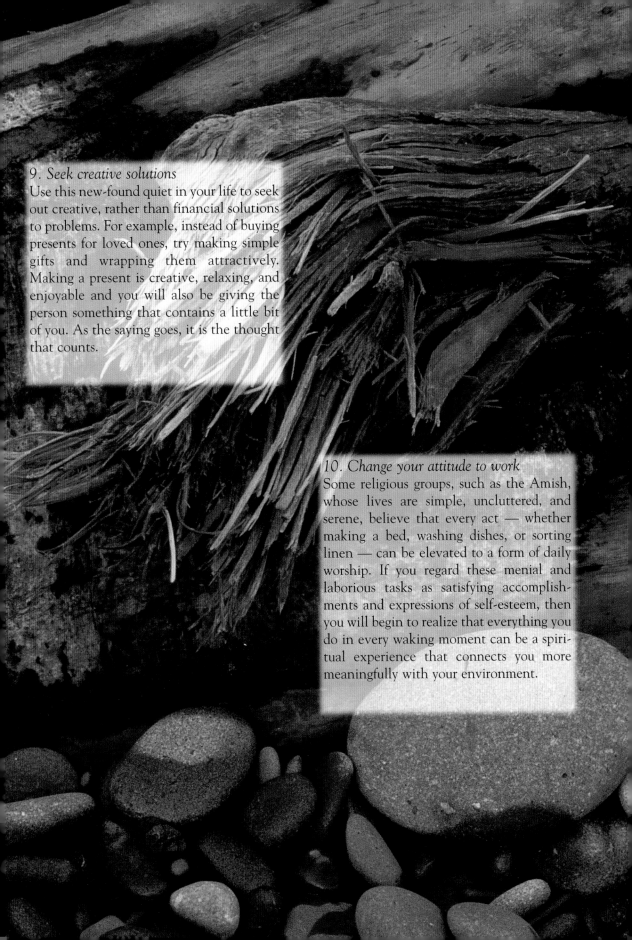

9. Seek creative solutions

Use this new-found quiet in your life to seek out creative, rather than financial solutions to problems. For example, instead of buying presents for loved ones, try making simple gifts and wrapping them attractively. Making a present is creative, relaxing, and enjoyable and you will also be giving the person something that contains a little bit of you. As the saying goes, it is the thought that counts.

10. Change your attitude to work

Some religious groups, such as the Amish, whose lives are simple, uncluttered, and serene, believe that every act — whether making a bed, washing dishes, or sorting linen — can be elevated to a form of daily worship. If you regard these menial and laborious tasks as satisfying accomplishments and expressions of self-esteem, then you will begin to realize that everything you do in every waking moment can be a spiritual experience that connects you more meaningfully with your environment.

Looking for Earth Signs

Nature, in the form of animals and birds, can offer you messages that become more evident the greater the balance of your own personal ecology. The shamanic world view sees the spirits of the animal kingdom as playing an important part in human life. Native Americans, for example, believe that an individual's power animal, or totem, acts as a signpost for their life, possessing certain qualities, offering guidance, protection, and helping with decision-making. Many pagan rituals involved wearing animal skins, dancing in the form of a certain creature, or calling upon the symbolic nature of the world of beasts — major or mini — to benefit an individual or tribe. Tai chi involves a series of movements mimicking a particular animal. Vision quests (see p.92) and sweat lodge ceremonies can help you to get in touch with your personal animal spirit guide. But the messages that Nature has for each of us can be gleaned from simply being aware of the animals, birds, feathers, and other omens that we come across in our daily lives.

Jane was standing in the kitchen looking out at her sacred space when she saw that a rabbit was nibbling at a bush. She had been distracted by sadness because her lover had left her. The assurance of an astrologer friend that he would be back in her life on or near the new Moon had failed to ease the pain. According to pagan belief, rabbits and hares have lunar associations and are considered good omens, symbolizing renewal. In Graeco-Roman traditions they were linked with Aphrodite, goddess of love, and were the companion of Cupid. That tranquil, but normally insignificant, sight of the rabbit filled her with hope and helped her focus on her work.

From today, be aware of any unusual happenings. Perhaps you will come across a feather lying in your path. Sacred objects like this are considered to be of great significance in esoteric terms, demonstrating a link with your Higher Self and your connection to the spirit world. You may see an animal, bird, or insect that you would not normally come across, or receive a card with an animal totem on it (see pp.108-9). Perhaps you might find yourself dreaming about a particular member of the animal kingdom or be drawn to a piece of jewellery or statue depicting one. Spirit animals not only have much to reveal about how we can live more spiritually fulfilling lives but they also act as a constant reminder that we are all part of the natural world.

We will then look at how you can achieve greater harmony in your home or workplace. However, the focus on what you can do to improve your personal ecology continues in Chapter Five, where there is a plethora of ways to further promote your physical, mental, emotional, and spiritual wellbeing.

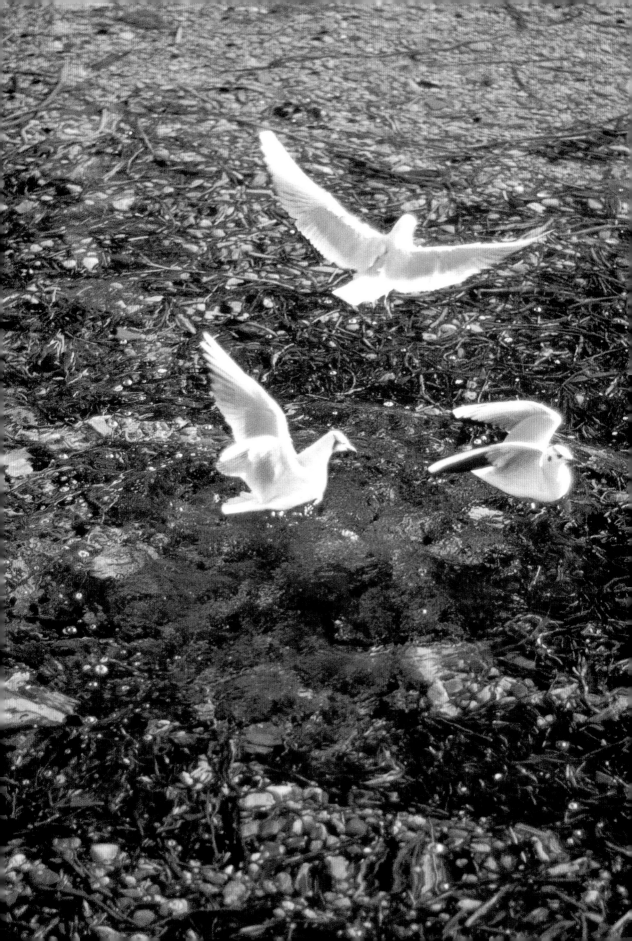

Personal Animal Totems

Pay attention to members of the animal kingdom you may come across in your daily life. They may have a message from the natural world to pass on to you.

Cuckoo *(herald of new fate)*

Trust your intuition — the instinctive knowledge within you that remains unexplained by reason or perception.

Cock *(watchfulness, resurrection)*

Be authentic and take greater delight in your authenticity, directness, enthusiasm, and humour.

Duck *(emotional comfort and protection)*

You may be paddling furiously through the emotions of your life, but allow the world to see your calmer side by assuming a grace with which to swim through these troubled waters. Everything is unfolding as it should.

Eagle *(healing and creativity)*

It's time to assume the power you have always been meant to demonstrate to the world. Tap in to your innate healing abilities and creativity.

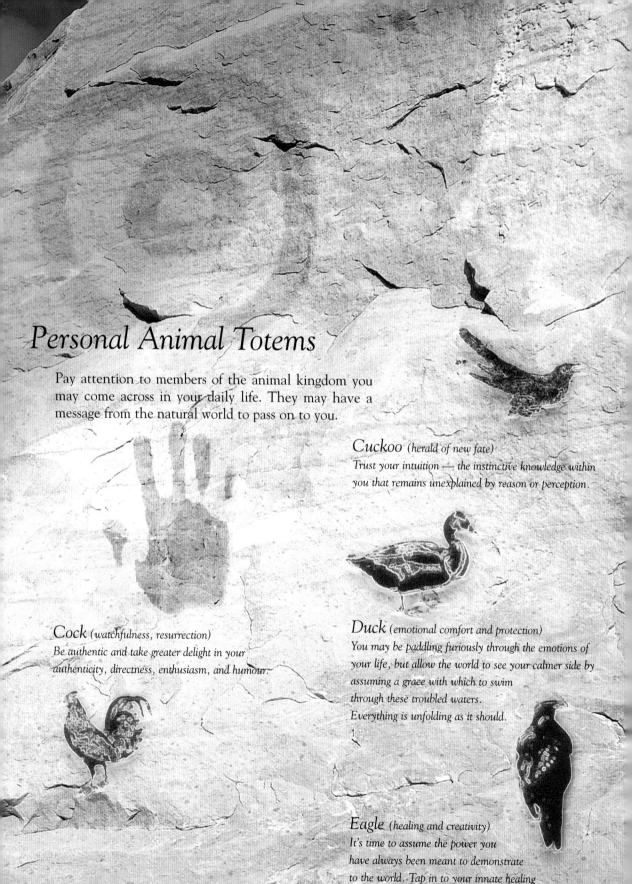

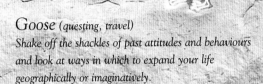

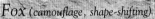

Goose (*questing, travel*)
Shake off the shackles of past attitudes and behaviours and look at ways in which to expand your life geographically or imaginatively.

Fox (*camouflage, shape-shifting*)
There is a need to develop new patterns of behaviour, even if they are not in line with how you think or feel. Take the action first and new thoughts will inevitably follow.

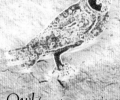

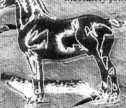

Owl (*mystery, magic, silent wisdom*)
Take more opportunity for silent meditation, to tune in to the hidden knowledge that you and others possess.

Horse (*power, freedom*)
In what ways are you restricting yourself? Is there something or someone you are holding on to that needs to be released in order for you to discover a greater freedom and power?

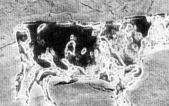

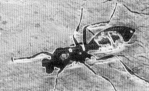

Bull (*fertility*)
What do you need to do to become more productive? What deeply rooted fears and behaviours may be preventing you from achieving more in your life?

Ant (*order, discipline*)
Success comes through effort now. Are you too obsessed with the "quick fix"? Be persistent and patient.

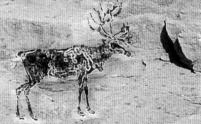

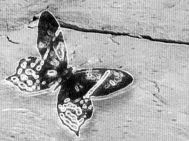

Deer (*gentleness, innocence*)
Be more gentle with yourself and others —in what new ways can you express unconditional love and enhance your life?

Butterfly (*transmutation*)
Lighten up and go with the flow. You may be resisting change, but it is an inevitable part of life. Look for the potential joy in new circumstances rather than the pain and trauma you habitually associate with change.

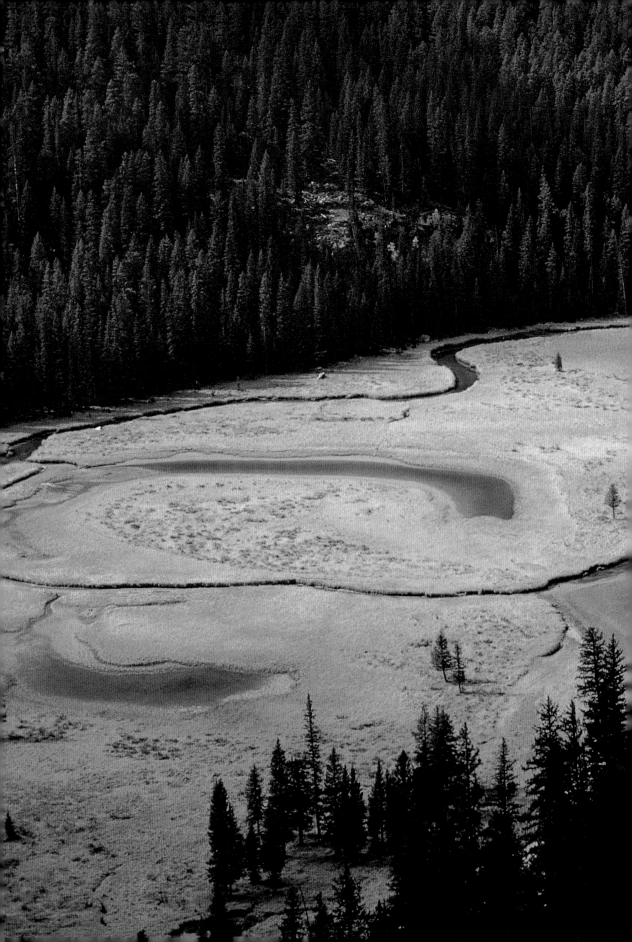

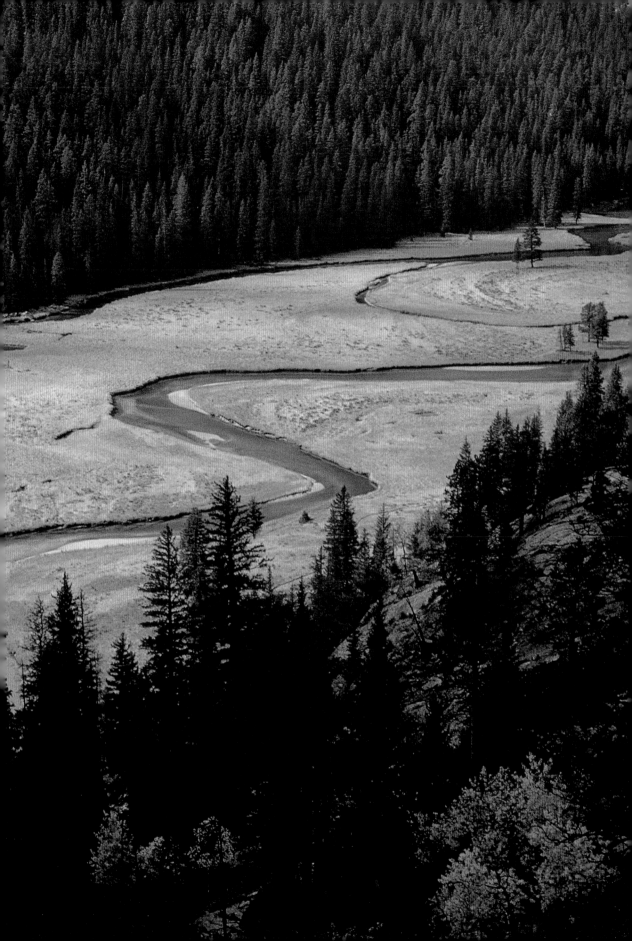

Your Home Environment

Many of us are familiar with the increasingly popular practice of feng shui, which, translated literally, means "wind and water" and acknowledges the auspicious nature of places where both of these elements flow smoothly. Long held in the East to be vital to health, wealth, and happiness this ancient practice of harmonious living has only recently become popular in the West. Despite seemingly complicated processes involving tools such as the Pa Kua, a special compass that indicates areas of good or bad energy in a place, the principle of feng shui is very simple: to be aware that there is an invisible world of energy that positively or negatively can affect human habitats and lives.

Less well known in the West is the Hindu equivalent of feng shui, vastu vidya, meaning "dwelling science". Like feng shui, this ancient practice offers practical ways in which to design, arrange, and organize your home or workplace and enhance your fortune and wellbeing. The forces of energy, or *gunas*, said to pervade all living areas fall into three categories, according to this system, and are required to be in balance. These are called Sattva (concentration of energy), Rajas (activity and diversity), and Tamas (chaos and entropy). Detecting which area is infused with which energy is undertaken — in a similar way to feng shui — by using an imaginary square, or Vastu Purusha, which is aligned with each of eight compass directions.

Both of these systems offer advice on how to remedy inauspicious locations. However, given that not everyone has the time, money, or desire to reposition walls or change the shape and size of rooms, it is important not to slavishly follow the rules laid down by these esoteric practices. Instead trust in your own intuition when deciding where to place furniture — particularly beds — which colour to paint walls, or where to position pictures and ornaments.

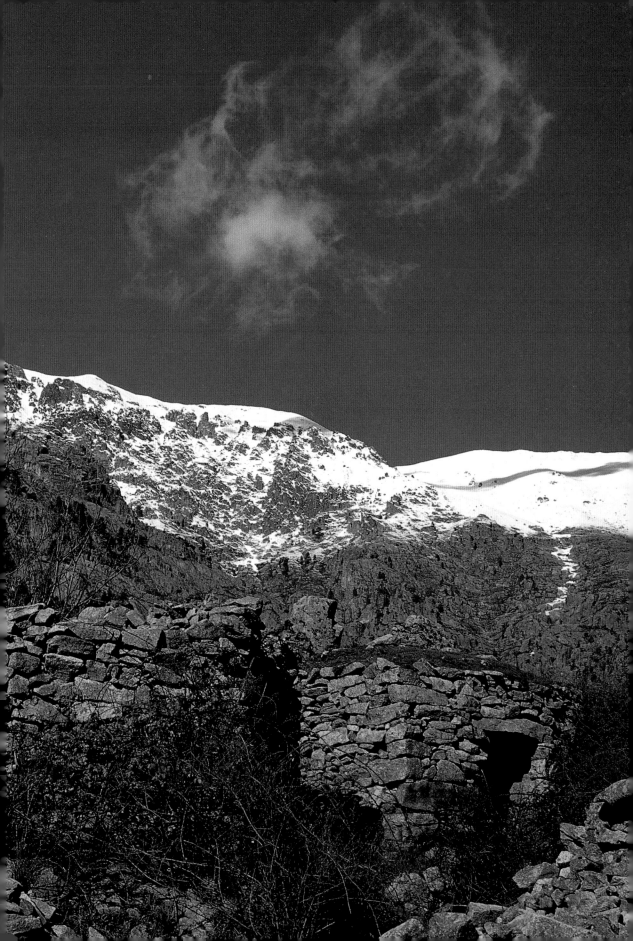

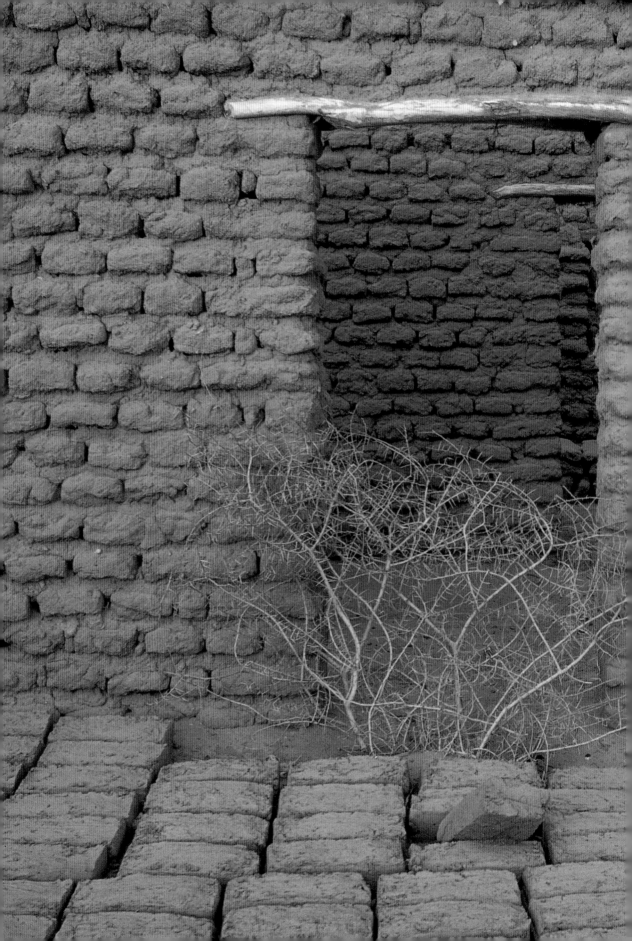

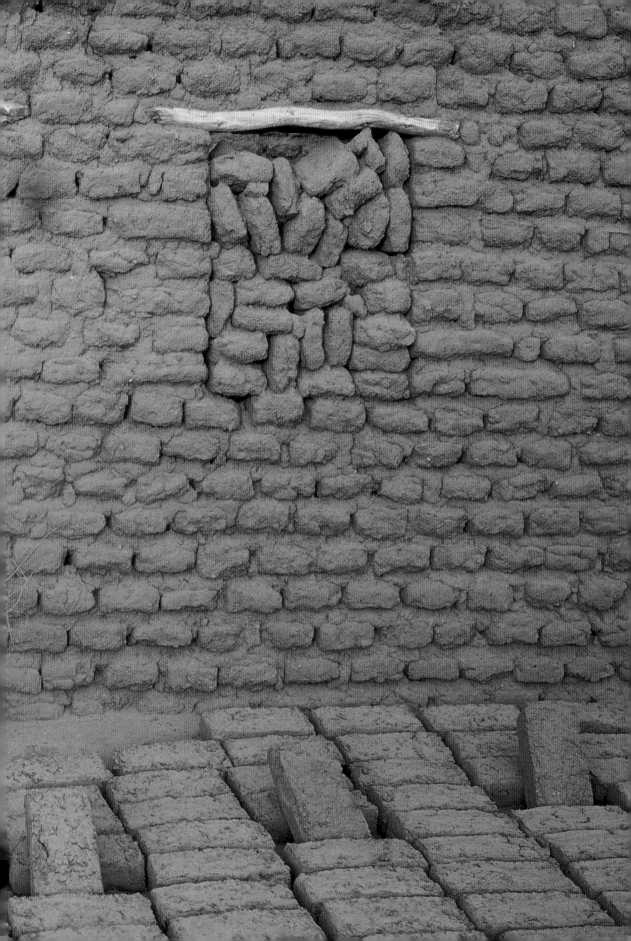

Room Cleansing 1

One practice that has developed from our Western fascination with Eastern geomantic systems like feng shui and vastu vidya is space clearing. Those of us who undertake regular "spring cleaning", irrespective of the time of year, are always aware of the enhanced energies of a room when it is clean and clutter-free. Yes, it looks better, but it also feels better in an ineffable way. The energy seems to flow more freely.

As with any spiritual activity it is essential to start out with a clear intention. As the saying goes "Where intention goes, energy flows". Perhaps you have been feeling under the weather recently for no medically detectable reason and wish to experience greater energy in your home or office. Or maybe your creativity has suffered and you want to do something to inject a bit of imaginative enterprise into your life. Perhaps your financial position seems to be stagnant and you would like to give that area of your life a kick start. Or it could be that you have determined to live in a more spiritually fulfilling way and want your environment to reflect that new focus.

Be clear about what you wish to achieve during this process and write down the specific results you expect to gain — in the short, medium, and long term. For example:

Intention: To enhance your innate creativity.

Area of Focus: The bedroom in which you write a nightly log of your day, or a spare room that you would like to turn into a studio for creative activities.

Goal(s):   To create a place where you can write the novel you have always had at the back of your mind and where you can engage in artistic activities (painting, making models, designing your garden, or dressmaking) instead of watching television (which for so many has become the "easy option" leisure activity).

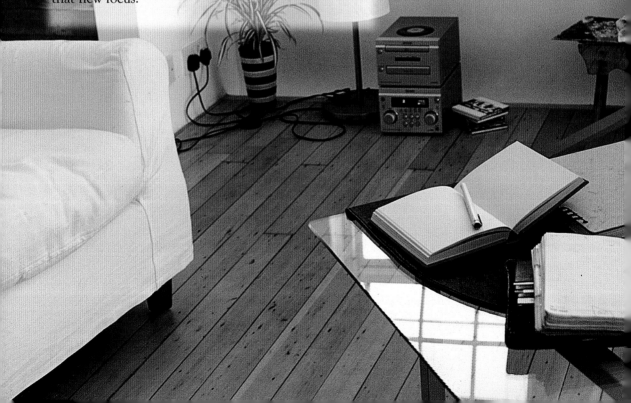

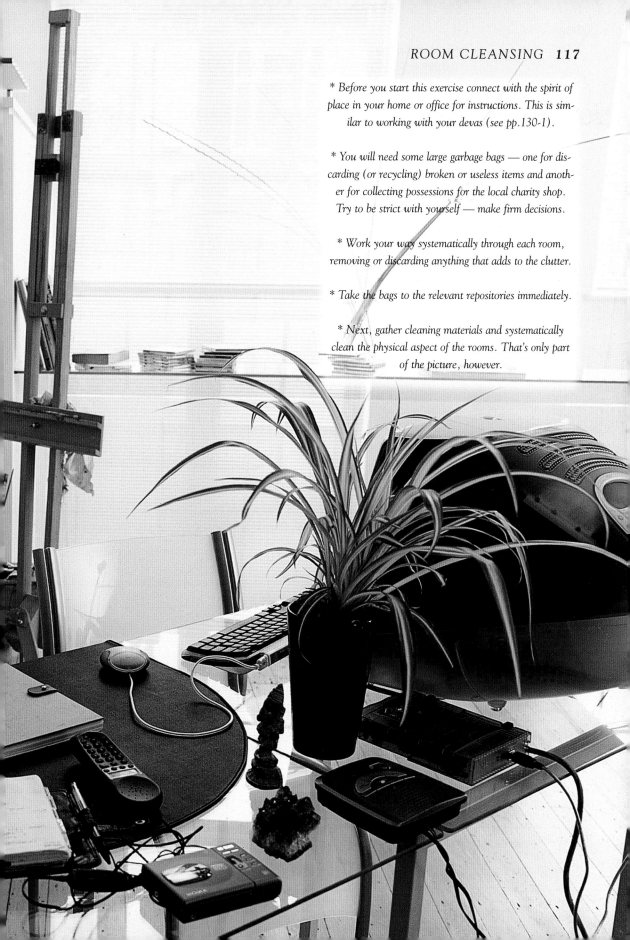

Before you start this exercise connect with the spirit of place in your home or office for instructions. This is similar to working with your devas (see pp.130-1).

You will need some large garbage bags — one for discarding (or recycling) broken or useless items and another for collecting possessions for the local charity shop. Try to be strict with yourself — make firm decisions.

Work your way systematically through each room, removing or discarding anything that adds to the clutter.

Take the bags to the relevant repositories immediately.

Next, gather cleaning materials and systematically clean the physical aspect of the rooms. That's only part of the picture, however.

Room Cleansing 2

Now think about the energetic cleansing that needs to take place on a regular basis in your home or work area. This kind of purification can take many forms, but the shamanic tradition of water purification, Native American smudging with smoking herbal sticks, and sound purification are the best and easiest to try out in the first instance.

Water purification

This involves flicking energized water from the end of a branch, twig, or with your fingertips around the room. Charge a bowl of water by leaving it in sunlight, moonlight, or placing a crystal in it for at least 24 hours. Be careful not to use crystals that are sensitive to water or are water-soluble, such as lapis lazuli, malachite, and turquoise. You might like to include an invocation as you perform this ritual, such as : "I ask the purifying energies of this water to cleanse this space and infuse it with love/light/healing/peace etc."

Smudging

This Native American custom has been used
for centuries in ceremonies in order to energeti-
cally cleanse a person or place. It is based on
the belief that exposing things to the smoke of
sacred fire or tobacco empowers them.
Commercial smudging sticks are usually made
of dried sage or a combination of sage and herbs
such as lemongrass or lavender.

1. Ignite one end of the sage stick and, after it
starts to burn, put out the flame and waft the
smoke around your body or the room. You can
use a feather to help direct the smoke if you
wish, or blow on it gently. Smudging purifies
the aura.

2. Ensure that your smudge stick is completely
extinguished at the end of your ceremony by
smothering the end with an old cloth, leaving it
outside on a safe ledge, or tapping the end
against a stone floor or in your garden.

Sound purification

Resonating sound is another excellent way of purifying
the energy of a room. Always choose a sound you like
— whether it's a Native American drum, bells, the
sound of clapping hands, or singing voices. Transmit the
sound throughout your room by walking around it —
paying special attention to the corners, in which stagnant
energy can become trapped.

Room Cleansing 3

The element of fire can be used to purify rooms and be linked with specific colours. Either buy a special long-burning candle, such as a church candle, which can be lit and left for several days at a time (with the proper precautions concerning children and pets) or smaller coloured or fragranced candles that relate to your specific intention and are burned for the day of cleansing only. Each of the rainbow colours is connected with a specific chakra, or energy centre, of the body. Similarly, the rooms in your home also have a different chakra connection. Hence, if you want to enhance the energy in a particular part of your home you should paint, decorate, or burn candles in the specific colour related to its corresponding chakra.

Red *(base or root chakra) for grounding and areas in which physical activity takes place, e.g. play rooms.*

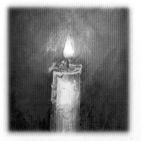

Green *(heart chakra) for unconditional love and tenderness and beneficial for any area in which the family spends time together, such as the sitting room.*

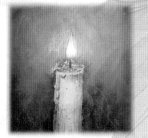

Blue *(throat chakra) for enhanced communication and self-expression, again useful for any areas used for art and creativity.*

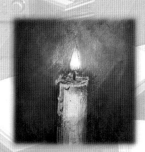

Orange (sacral chakra) for creativity, sensuality, and emotional balance, e.g. a study or bedrooms.

Yellow (solar plexus chakra) linked with the digestive system, this colour is particularly good for burning in dining rooms and kitchens.

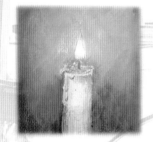

Purple/Indigo (third eye chakra) to enhance psychic awareness and intuition, therefore good for meditation areas, sacred spaces, and altars.

White/Gold (crown chakra) combines all the chakras and is therefore perfect for burning throughout your home or office. Connected with the Higher Self and enlightenment — the perfection of mind, body, and spirit.

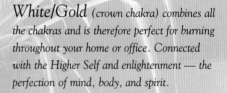

Dowsing for Sick-Building Syndrome

The Earth produces negative energies that have been identified with geopathic stress, which is also thought to be the cause of "sick-building syndrome" (SBS), resulting in manifestations such as headaches, fatigue, and cold or flu-like symptoms. One study has found that 90 per cent of staff in all offices investigated suffer from some signs of SBS. The causes of SBS are thought to be related to both the electromagnetic fields generated by high-tech equipment, computers, power cables, lights, and other electrical equipment, playing havoc with the human immune system, plus the radiation coming from blocked underground streams, as "black streams", amplified by the metal frames of modern office buildings.

To identify which areas of your home or office are concentrated centres for geopathic stress, you may wish to contact a dowser. However, you can identify these health-threatening areas yourself.

1. Make a set of dowsing rods (see pp.86-7).

2. Hold them lightly in your hands, as shown, and walk slowly but steadily around the room.

3. You will know when you have come across a stress line because the rods will suddenly swing outward or inward and cross each other.

4. Check the area several times, perhaps at different times of day or with another person, to ensure that it is terrestrial electromagnetism that's influencing the rods and not your own movements.

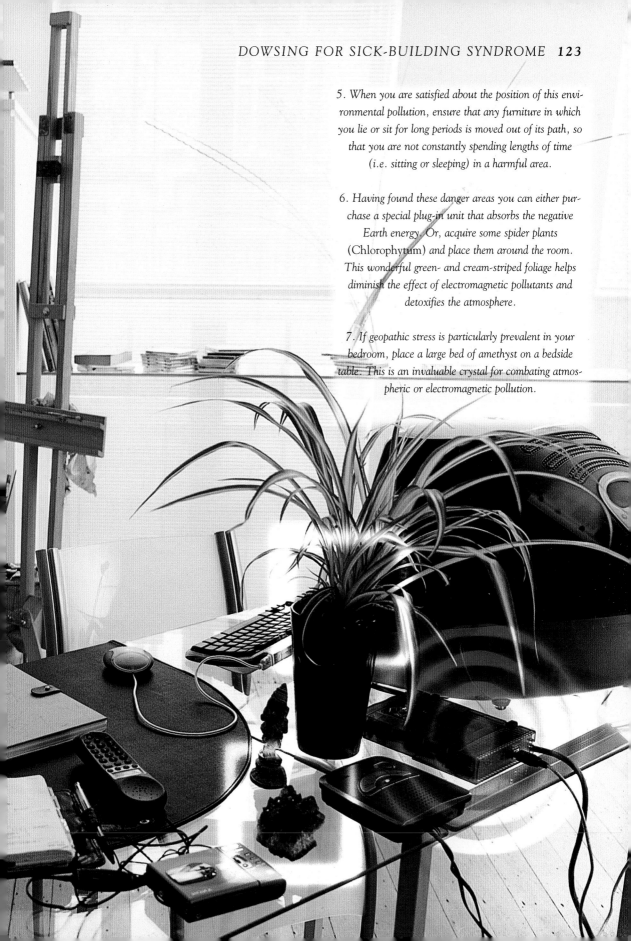

5. When you are satisfied about the position of this environmental pollution, ensure that any furniture in which you lie or sit for long periods is moved out of its path, so that you are not constantly spending lengths of time (i.e. sitting or sleeping) in a harmful area.

6. Having found these danger areas you can either purchase a special plug-in unit that absorbs the negative Earth energy. Or, acquire some spider plants (Chlorophytum) and place them around the room. This wonderful green- and cream-striped foliage helps diminish the effect of electromagnetic pollutants and detoxifies the atmosphere.

7. If geopathic stress is particularly prevalent in your bedroom, place a large bed of amethyst on a bedside table. This is an invaluable crystal for combating atmospheric or electromagnetic pollution.

Your Outdoor Environment

Your garden or outdoor space offers a very obvious means of connecting with Earth. A colourful, healthy, outdoor environment, abundant with flowers, vegetables, herbs, insects, and other small creatures, is a tangible expression of energetic balance. Unfortunately, humankind has become overly obsessed with manufactured products that supposedly encourage our gardens to grow and kill all the insect "pests" that interfere with our efforts. Such is the proliferation of insecticides and fertilizers that it now seems incredible that we ever managed to feed ourselves for so many millennia without them. Yet, as horticulturalists point out, undisturbed Mother Nature maintains perfect control: the more balanced, in terms of the diversification of plants, that your garden is, the more it will naturally attract predators such as ladybirds that eat up flower-consuming aphids and other pests (see pp.126-7).

Modern education systems, particularly within the scientific community, advocate specialization, discouraging, for example, the study of art and science together and thereby precluding the opportunity to view life holistically. This is diametrically opposed to the sort of approach that produced polymath geniuses such as Einstein, Da Vinci, and Edison. Similarly, concentrating on one or two crops to the exclusion of others, which, in rotation, would replenish the Earth with vital nutrients, has been the cause of poor yields in the past and necessitated the use of commercially produced fertilizers. However, dealing with the effects of bad harvests, while failing to understand and tackle underlying causes, is not just short-sighted but environmentally irresponsible.

Crop specialization is not a modern phenomenon: during the thirteenth century horticultural ignorance contributed to the degradation and exhaustion of English soils, which resulted in terrible famines. These set the scene for the Black Death that ravaged almost half the population of the UK in the fourteenth century. Because of the devastating loss of available farm labour, crop farming was significantly reduced, to be replaced by pastureland, and sheep grazing. Our medieval ancestors may have used a simple method of crop rotation, leaving one area fallow for a year, but that did not offer enough diversification or time for the soil to recover fully. It was only after a century of rest and of fertilizing the soil with readily available rotting grass and sheep's manure that England's soils were healthy enough to resume arable farming. However, it was only when Thomas Coke of Holkham (1776-1816) introduced his high-yielding, four-course rotational system — turnips, barley, clover, followed by wheat — did farmers begin to use an approach more in keeping with the natural cycle of return. The Chinese have intensively farmed their lands for thousands of years, often producing three crops annually, but because of their understanding of composting and the need to return wastes to the land, they have successfully fed the population, without soil exhaustion.

Unless we wish to be force-fed an unpleasant diet of laboratory-engineered foods that are subject to irradiation and genetic modification, then we must recognize that our future depends on Earth's ability to feed us. Gaia is perfectly capable of this, provided we all play our part in assisting her. Whether you choose to grow your own produce or not, in your own small way you can encourage the proliferation of plants that attract predatory birds and beneficial insects. By growing plants that compliment each other, by planting bedding fruit, vegetables, flowers, and herbs together rather than in rigidly specialized plots, by choosing strains known to be strong and disease-resistant, you will provide the best conditions for Nature to do her work.

We may not like the fact that plant-eating insects exist in the mini-beast world, but they are part of Nature's clean-up squad. These creatures attack only sick or dying plants — it is believed they do so by using their antennae to sense the plants' intensified infrared light pulses — in order to help recycle the waste back into the ground. By and large healthy plants do not attract insect attacks.

The Positive Role of Pests

Here are a few examples of the important role that different so-called pests play in the ecology of this planet.

Wasps

Adult wasps, being largely carnivorous, feed on other insects and their remains, including destructive caterpillars that destroy commercial crops. One species of wasp native to Africa eats rhinoceros beetle eggs, an insect that destroys coconuts and detrimentally affects the economy of those regions. However, wasps also dispose of overripe vegetable matter, contributing to life's natural waste-disposal cycle.

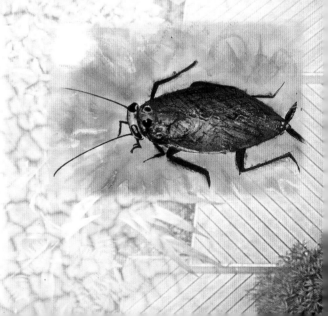

Flies

Despite being associated largely with disease and unpleasantness, these insects also play an important role in nature's balancing act. They speed up the decomposition of animal and vegetable matter that would otherwise fester for much longer. They prey on other insects and are responsible for the culling and control of some more harmful species. Flies also carry pollen to plants.

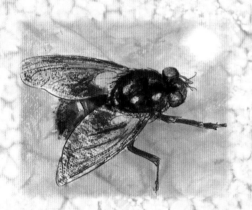

Cockroaches

Another important player in Earth's ecosystem, these rather unpleasant-looking insects, like flies, assist the fast decomposition of decaying plants and animal faeces. They provide food for many animals (including human beings in some parts of the world) and are interesting to study in the laboratory because they are remarkably resistant and adaptive to all the pesticides that humankind sprays on them. Considering that cockroaches have lived on this planet for at least 320 million years, there is, potentially, much we can learn from them.

Other friends to the gardener, helping to control pests, include: black-kneed capsids, centipedes, ground beetles, hover flies, harvestmen (long-legged "spiders"), lacewings, ladybirds, and spiders.

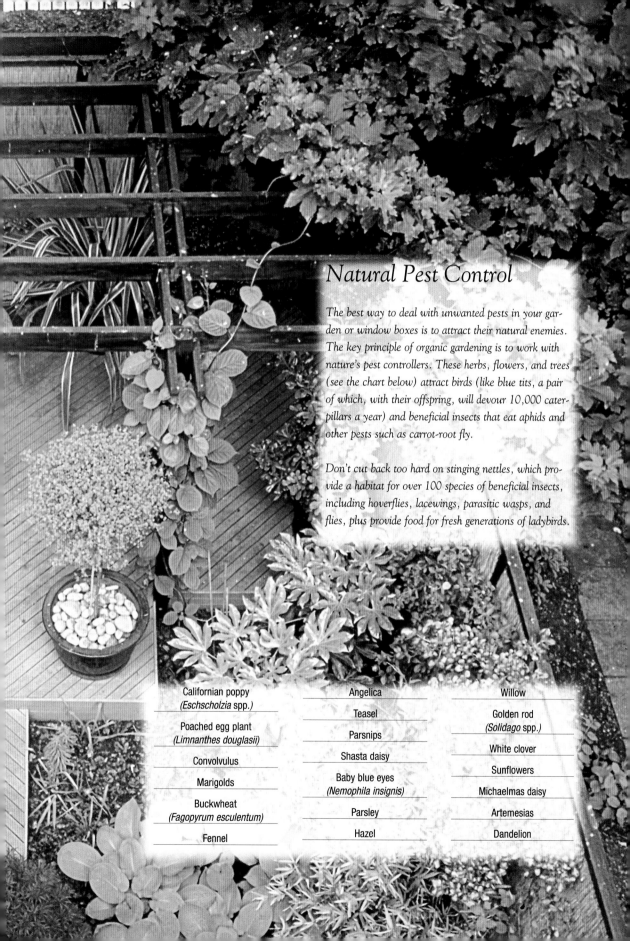

Natural Pest Control

The best way to deal with unwanted pests in your garden or window boxes is to attract their natural enemies. The key principle of organic gardening is to work with nature's pest controllers. These herbs, flowers, and trees (see the chart below) attract birds (like blue tits, a pair of which, with their offspring, will devour 10,000 caterpillars a year) and beneficial insects that eat aphids and other pests such as carrot-root fly.

Don't cut back too hard on stinging nettles, which provide a habitat for over 100 species of beneficial insects, including hoverflies, lacewings, parasitic wasps, and flies, plus provide food for fresh generations of ladybirds.

Californian poppy (*Eschscholzia* spp.)	Angelica	Willow
Poached egg plant (*Limnanthes douglasii*)	Teasel	Golden rod (*Solidago* spp.)
Convolvulus	Parsnips	White clover
Marigolds	Shasta daisy	Sunflowers
Buckwheat (*Fagopyrum esculentum*)	Baby blue eyes (*Nemophila insignis*)	Michaelmas daisy
Fennel	Parsley	Artemesias
	Hazel	Dandelion

Gardening Action

You can play your part in ecological recycling in the following ways:

Composting

Compost as much household and garden waste as possible, including fruit and vegetable peelings, overripe fruit, horse manure, paper, weeds (minus the seed heads), grass clippings, and fallen leaves. Place them in a commercial composter or set aside a small corner of your garden to allow natural decomposition to take place. Throw in a quantity of nettles, which act as natural activators in the process.

Avoid chemicals

Cut down, or avoid altogether, the use of chemical herbicides, pesticides, and fertilizers. It was only many years after the introduction of products such as DDT that they were found to leave toxic residues in the soil, kill beneficial insects as well as unwanted ones, poison wildlife, infect the food chain, and contribute to the dying out of many species. DDT is held responsible for the thinning out of the shells of some birds of prey, including falcons, causing many generations of eggs to fail to hatch. Many of the chemicals brought on to the market in the 1950s and 1960s have subsequently been banned because of their carcinogenic links and the ways in which they damage the natural environment.

Recycling

Lobby your local government to do more to encourage recycling. Apart from the usual bottle banks and reuse sites, Holland and Germany have established many large composting centres where household, organic waste — collected from homes on a weekly basis — is used to replenish the soil. In some areas of Holland, householders are further encouraged to take part in these schemes by being paid, by weight, for the amount of recyclable organic waste they contribute.

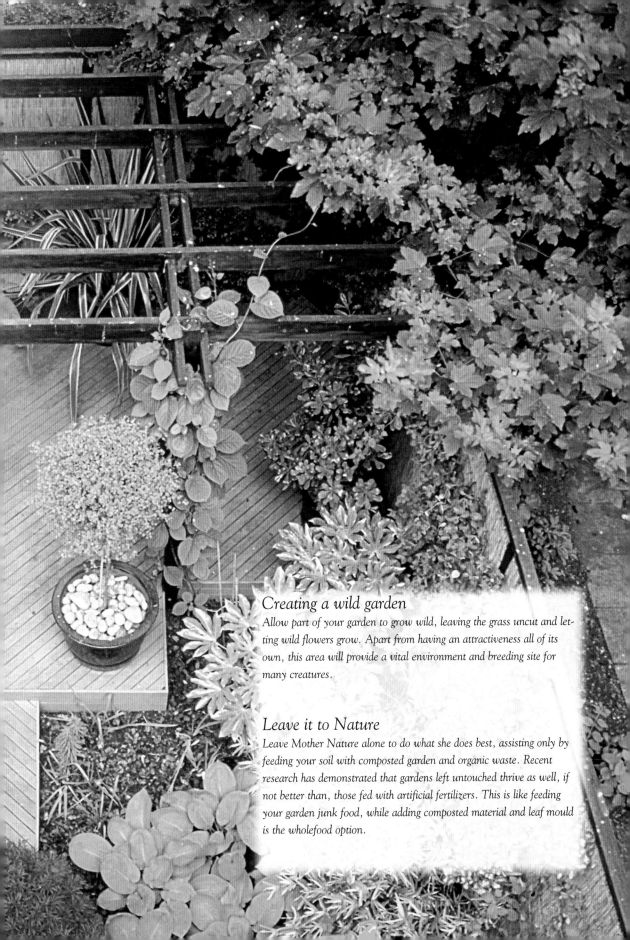

Creating a wild garden

Allow part of your garden to grow wild, leaving the grass uncut and letting wild flowers grow. Apart from having an attractiveness all of its own, this area will provide a vital environment and breeding site for many creatures.

Leave it to Nature

Leave Mother Nature alone to do what she does best, assisting only by feeding your soil with composted garden and organic waste. Recent research has demonstrated that gardens left untouched thrive as well, if not better than, those fed with artificial fertilizers. This is like feeding your garden junk food, while adding composted material and leaf mould is the wholefood option.

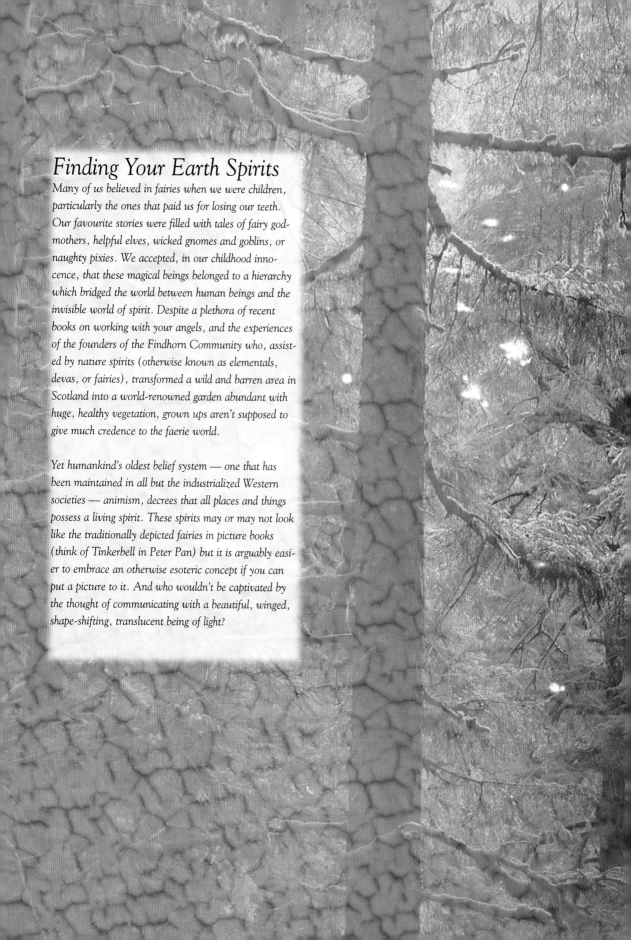

Finding Your Earth Spirits

Many of us believed in fairies when we were children, particularly the ones that paid us for losing our teeth. Our favourite stories were filled with tales of fairy godmothers, helpful elves, wicked gnomes and goblins, or naughty pixies. We accepted, in our childhood innocence, that these magical beings belonged to a hierarchy which bridged the world between human beings and the invisible world of spirit. Despite a plethora of recent books on working with your angels, and the experiences of the founders of the Findhorn Community who, assisted by nature spirits (otherwise known as elementals, devas, or fairies), transformed a wild and barren area in Scotland into a world-renowned garden abundant with huge, healthy vegetation, grown ups aren't supposed to give much credence to the faerie world.

Yet humankind's oldest belief system — one that has been maintained in all but the industrialized Western societies — animism, decrees that all places and things possess a living spirit. These spirits may or may not look like the traditionally depicted fairies in picture books (think of Tinkerbell in Peter Pan) but it is arguably easier to embrace an otherwise esoteric concept if you can put a picture to it. And who wouldn't be captivated by the thought of communicating with a beautiful, winged, shape-shifting, translucent being of light?

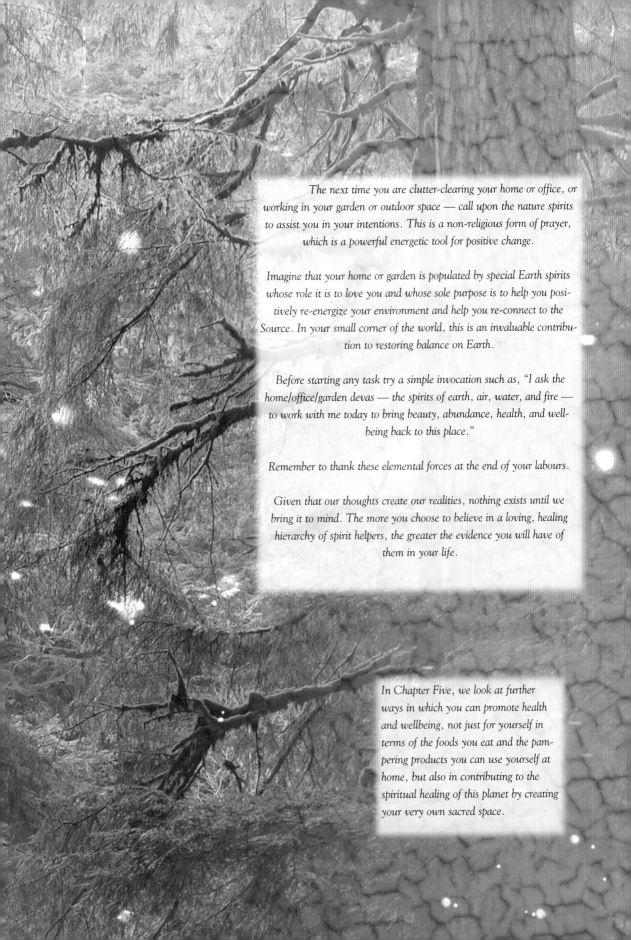

The next time you are clutter-clearing your home or office, or working in your garden or outdoor space — call upon the nature spirits to assist you in your intentions. This is a non-religious form of prayer, which is a powerful energetic tool for positive change.

Imagine that your home or garden is populated by special Earth spirits whose role it is to love you and whose sole purpose is to help you positively re-energize your environment and help you re-connect to the Source. In your small corner of the world, this is an invaluable contribution to restoring balance on Earth.

Before starting any task try a simple invocation such as, "I ask the home/office/garden devas — the spirits of earth, air, water, and fire — to work with me today to bring beauty, abundance, health, and wellbeing back to this place."

Remember to thank these elemental forces at the end of your labours.

Given that our thoughts create our realities, nothing exists until we bring it to mind. The more you choose to believe in a loving, healing hierarchy of spirit helpers, the greater the evidence you will have of them in your life.

In Chapter Five, we look at further ways in which you can promote health and wellbeing, not just for yourself in terms of the foods you eat and the pampering products you can use yourself at home, but also in contributing to the spiritual healing of this planet by creating your very own sacred space.

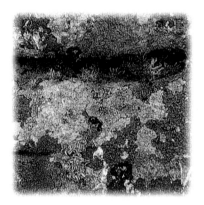

This Healing Earth

In our society of convenience, where services are becoming increasingly available at the click of a button, we have come to expect instant cures for illness and minor complaints, typically in a bottle of pills, at the end of a needle, or under a laser beam. In the wake of modern technology it is easy to forget that Nature offers a rich source of remedies for the body, mind, and spirit, which work without the side-effects often associated with conventional medicine.

We will begin this chapter by exploring Nature's pharmacy and consider some of the latest research into the benefits of phyto-medicines — those derived from plants — for health and healing. We will then examine how these medicines can be taken internally as food supplements, for example, and used externally, suggesting how mineral salts, fruits, plants, and soils can be incorporated into your beauty regime. We will also consider the healing properties of crystals and how their natural frequencies can re-establish your body's optimum health.

Finally, drawing together the concepts introduced in this book, we will discuss how you can create your own sacred space. A place, whether it be as small as a window box or as extensive as any garden — where you can regularly tune in to the healing energies of Earth.

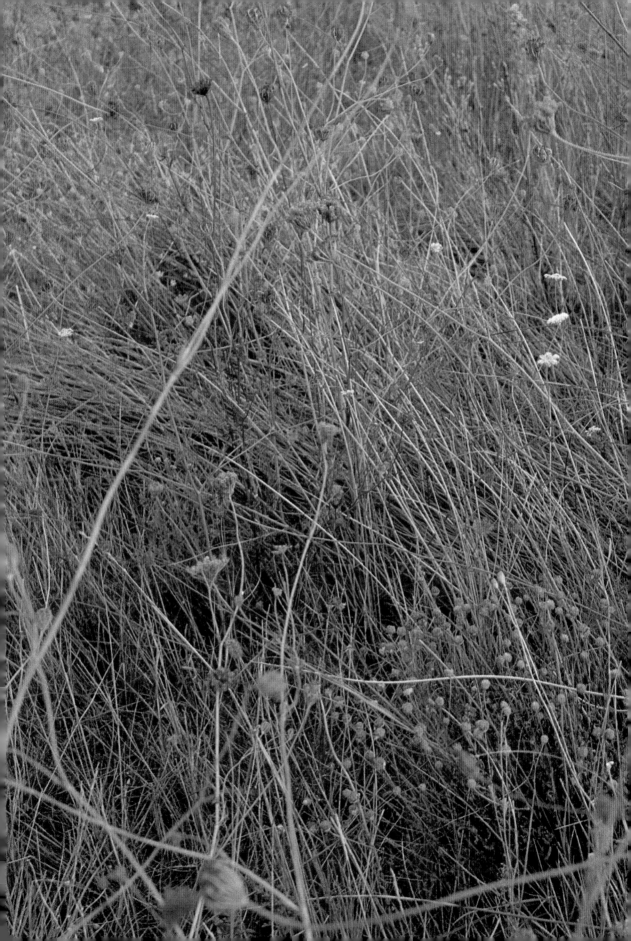

Nature's Pharmacy

For centuries people have sought medical advice or
treatment from physicians or healers. Where we now
take medicines orally, healing in the past often involved
the imbibing or rubbing in of a plant-based medicine, or
on a more spiritual level, the laying on of hands or
prayer. The patient's role, particularly in the West, has
always been a predominantly passive one, handing over
the responsibility for our recovery to a greater authority,
one whose medical qualifications or supernatural powers
are widely respected. This attitude, though still prevalent, is changing: faced with a life-threatening illness, or
even a relatively minor one, more of us are taking
responsibility for ourselves, finding out how our bodies
work, what we need to do to maintain optimum health,
whether manufactured drugs will cause us greater damage than our original complaints, and how changing the
way we think will have a direct bearing on what happens
to us physically. More importantly, increasing numbers
of us are doing this before illness strikes. This is a major
paradigm shift for Western societies that have hitherto
promoted disease care rather than health care. Why wait
to become ill when, with knowledge, application, and
dedication, we can prevent illness and live longer,
healthier, and happier lives?

Centuries ago, though this tradition persists in some
societies, it was the shaman, witch doctor, or wise
woman who administered plant-based concoctions to
effect a cure. Today we can go to a health-food store, buy
organic food, and seek advice from therapists or books to
learn how to promote our own good health. With the
aid of modern technology we are beginning to discover
how specific plant constituents — phytochemicals —
work to protect, repair, and heal us.

A Return to Folk Medicine

This health awareness is both essential and timely as
concerns surrounding the link between high levels of
pesticides, herbicides, and degenerative diseases esca-
late. It is no longer enough to eat a well-balanced diet

when essential nutrients in the soil are being depleted by intensive farming practices and when the impact of irradiated and genetically modified food has yet to be fully appreciated. Recent food scares, such as the BSE ("mad cow" disease) crisis in the UK, have also prompted people to consider more seriously what they eat and how this has an impact on their health. Incidences of stroke, cancers, and rheumatoid arthritis are all on the increase, many cases of which could be avoided, if not alleviated, through informed, nutritional approaches.

The benefits of traditional folk medicine, based on the healing powers of plants, were largely lost to us once medical science and big businesses began to dominate health care. While this knowledge is currently being rediscovered and repackaged to suit a more discriminating consumer, this shift in treatment is slow and not without its opponents and cynics. However, they should not exaggerate the extent to which recent advances in medical science have prolonged and enhanced our lives, for the average life expectancy in the West has risen by only two years since the 1920s. Why modern medicine has not extended our life spans further can be explained in part by its general approach to health care: it focuses primarily on treating the symptoms of an illness rather than its cause, often suppressing a condition that later re-emerges as a more serious illness, or causing side-effects more distressing to the patient than the original condition. Perhaps it is time for the West to review its general approach to medicine.

Many researchers are indeed turning back to nature for answers: in the USA, for example, scientists have produced a non-toxic version of viper venom, which, when given to 500 stroke patients, dissolved blood clots sufficiently for them to recover their physical and mental capabilities within three hours of an attack; in Germany and the USA researchers have found that a natural antioxidant called pycnogenol, extracted from pine tree bark, helps protect against heart disease, stroke, and premature ageing; it may even play an important part in preventing inflammatory diseases.

Hippocrates was right, over 2,000 years ago, when he said, "Let food be your medicine and medicine your food". Known as the father of medicine from whose name the contemporary medical profession takes its Hippocratic oath, the Greek physician taught his students to treat the whole person, not just the disease, to consider lifestyle and habits, and to encourage the innate capacity of the human body to heal itself. This holistic approach can still be seen in modern homeopathy and other alternative practices, modern orthodox medicine being more inclined to isolate the symptoms. Ironically Hippocrates' treatments, which included massage with essential oils, hydrotherapy, plenty of fresh air and sunlight, exercise, and wholesome food, were so effective that the philosopher Plato complained that people were living too long. Such regimes became increasingly popular throughout Greece and Rome, inspiring later physicians such as Dioscorides and Galen to formulate and record hundreds of medicinal plant cures for countless ailments.

Unfortunately it seems that many of these ancient remedies fell into the hands of opportunistic apothecaries, who, over the centuries, manipulated the original formulations and charged high prices. Gradually Hippocrates's philosophy of relying on Nature's healing force to cure illness was forgotten, particularly with the development of organic chemistry in the eighteenth and nineteenth centuries.

Even when modern medicine uses plants as a base for new drugs by synthetically producing the active constituents of plants, the impurities or apparently non-active constituents of a plant, which often play an essential role in assisting and easing the absorption of natural plant chemicals in the body, are lost. These additional ingredients can also protect against exceeding the body's tolerance levels of any one particular compound, thereby mitigating otherwise unpleasant side-effects. For example, ephedrine, isolated from the Chinese herb, *Ephedra sinica*, was once marketed as a drug for asthma.

By itself, the chemical was found to raise blood pressure to dangerous levels and has consequently been largely withdrawn from circulation. However, in its crude form, this plant has been used in China for thousands of years with no harmful side-effects. The pharmaceutical industry's reluctance to promote natural remedies can be better understood in terms of economics: botanic medicines cannot be patented, whereas synthetic drugs can. It is these patented medicines that earn companies vast sums of money, regardless of the fact that synthetic drugs are unable fully to replicate the effects of the equivalent natural plant medicine and are not as easily absorbed into the human body.

Nature's pharmacy is impressive for the range of conditions to which it can be applied. There is so much more to plants than providing us with essential vitamins, minerals, and trace elements. Tests carried out on phyto, or plant, chemicals are illuminating: allicin, found in garlic, onions, and leeks, lowers blood cholesterol and protects against many cancers; alpha carotene in carrots and seaweed boosts the immune system; beta carotene, found in dark green, red, and yellow vegetables and fruits, reduces the risk of numerous cancers; lycopene in red and orange fruits such as apricots, red grapefruit, and tomatoes protects against age-related cell damage; tannins found in certain plants such as willow, witch-hazel, and oak, have astringent and antiseptic properties that help diarrhoea, mouth infections, and slow-healing wounds; and one group of natural chemicals, called triterpenoid saponins — found in ginseng and wild yam — act as precursors to the sex hormones. Fortunately, with a greater scientific understanding of plants and natural remedies, it is becoming increasingly common to use a honey-based syrup as a cough remedy or vinegar and lemon to soothe a wasp sting — just as it was before manufactured drugs became more widely available. Not so much old wives' tales, but old, wise advice.

Living Foods

The following chart lists a number of common foods and herbs, with their active constituents and corresponding healing properties. Try to include as many of them in your diet as possible (preferably organically grown), to avoid many degenerative diseases:

NAME	ACTIVE CONSTITUENTS	MEDICINAL USES
Cranberry juice	Anthocyanins	Helps stop bacteria attaching to the bladder, thereby preventing and alleviating urinary-tract infections.
Licorice	Triterpenoids; glycyrrhizin	Anti-tumour properties; boosts immune system; fights gum disease and tooth decay; improves liver function.
Green tea	Catechins	Lowers cholesterol levels; boosts body's metabolic rate and believed to boost immune system; protects against some cancers and premature ageing.
Soya milk & tofu	Genistein; phyto-oestrogens	Particularly valuable to women in protection against breast cancer, osteoporosis, menstrual and menopausal disorders, and hormone-related diseases. Also lowers cholesterol.
Berries (e.g. strawberries)	Flavonoids	Strengthen blood capillaries; speed up healing of wounds, sprains, and muscle injuries. Improve the body's ability to absorb and utilize vitamin C.
Oily fish (e.g. sardines and mackerel)	Co-enzyme Q10	Plays important role in balancing the body's metabolic rate; helps normalize blood pressure; boosts immunity; improves heart functioning and tolerance to exercise.
Olive oil	Glycerides of oleic acid	Taken internally (1 tablespoon first thing in the morning), treatment for constipation; externally, said to be a natural sunscreen, filtering up to 20 per cent of sun's rays.
Peppermint	Essential oils, flavonoids, carotenoids, etc.	Anti-inflammatory, antiseptic, and anti-spasmodic properties. Drunk as tea, for indigestion, diarrhoea, flatulence, and stomach pains. Said to aid healing of gastric ulcers.
Lavender	Essential oils, tannins, and flavonoids	Natural sedative and anti-depressant, useful taken as a weak infusion for nervous disorders, insomnia, and irritability. Externally cooled infusions can treat vaginal infections, cuts and sores, insect stings, and minor burns.
Cauliflower, Brussels sprouts	Sulforaphane, isothiocyanates, and indoles	Assists in the detoxification of cells to aid cancer-fighting and anti-ageing enzymes. Research suggests that more than one portion of brassica weekly will reduce the risk of developing cancer of the colon by two-thirds.
Ginger	Gingerol (combination of volatile oils and resin)	Anti-inflammatory properties prohibit and block the production of compounds that increase swelling and cause pain in conditions such as rheumatism, osteoarthritis, and migraines. Also anti-emetic, good as tea for motion and morning sickness, nausea and vomiting. Also possesses beneficial properties for treatment of heartburn, abdominal cramps, and poor digestion.

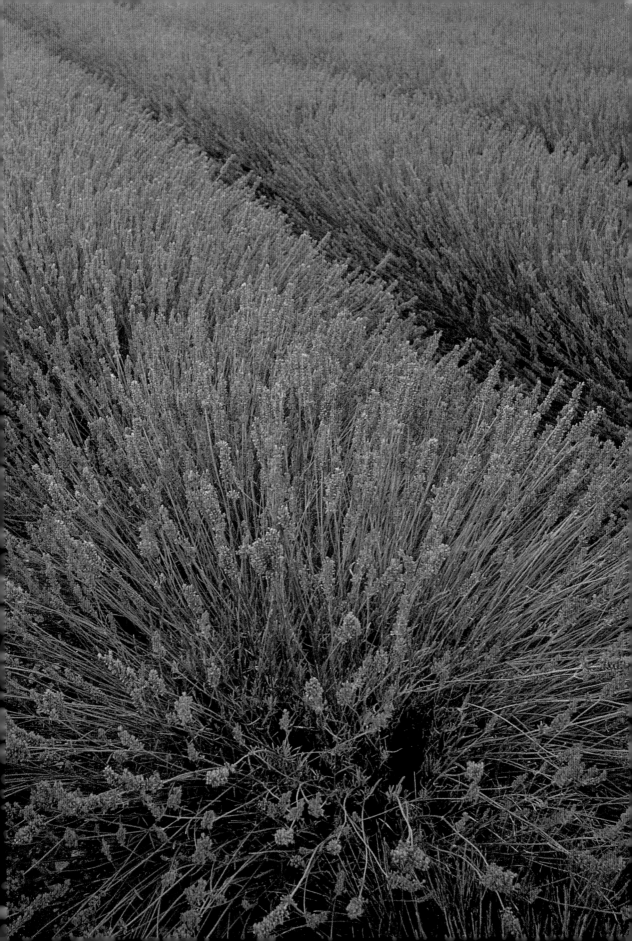

Energy Medicine

However, the beneficial properties of plants extend beyond their immediately detectable biochemical healing properties: plants, like all living species, resonate energies that can heal the body. Homeopathy and Bach Flower Remedies work on this principle, though the orthodox medical profession rejects their validity because, on chemical analysis, there appears to be no active constituent left. Rooted in the biochemical domain, the influence of physics is often overlooked.

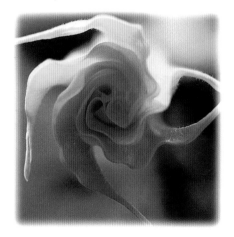

The "soul like" properties of natural substances were of particular fascination to Swiss German physician and alchemist, Paracelsus (1493-1541). Having studied medical science in Italy, Paracelsus (ironically perceived as the founder of the pharmaceutical chemistry) rejected his orthodox education, preferring to focus on the compatible resonances between physician, patient, and plants. He believed in "cosmic correspondences", whereby the colours of plants — colour simply being an indicator of differing frequencies, shape, or likeness to a particular part of the human body — are indicative of their healing properties.

Two hundred years before the German doctor, Samuel Hahnemann, founded modern homeopathy, Paracelsus was announcing that diluted natural substances administered in minute amounts would cure diseases with which they had a natural energetic affinity. It is for this reason that homeopaths pay great attention to a person's mental and emotional condition, as well as their physical history, in order to prescribe a remedy to overcome their disharmony holistically, and not just in terms of the particular symptoms that are currently affecting them. Hahnemann's system of medicine was inspired by the discovery that the herbal remedy for malaria, cinchona tree bark, would produce the symptoms of that disease — including fever and headache — when taken by a healthy person, but would cure someone suffering from malaria. The rationale behind this was that such symptoms were the body's natural way of fighting illness, so that any medicine that provoked the same symptoms would aid recovery. Later, quinine was isolated from cinchona bark and became the first anti-malaria drug.

The energetic life force that courses through all things has many names. In Indian traditions it is called prana whereas the Ancient Chinese referred to it as chi. Even orthodox science acknowledges that there is a bioelectromagnetic field in all life, while resisting the notion that this has a major part to play in health and healing. This energy field can be seen by some individuals, who call it the aura, but it can also be detected and even photographed by special machinery such as that developed by the Russian researcher, Semyon Kirlian, in the 1930s. Pioneering work conducted by neurophysiologist and psychologist, Dr Valerie V. Hunt, based on NASA space technology, is leading us to a greater scientific understanding of how the energetic frequencies of plants, minerals, and other natural agents help to balance and thereby cure dysfunctional vibrations within our body cells.

This continuous, electromagnetic radiation from the atomic matter of all things, animate and inanimate, allows for an exchange of energy between individuals and plant or mineral life, and is the reasoning behind the benefits of crystal healing (see pp.146-7). Similarly, when you take a homeopathic preparation or a few drops of Bach Flower Remedy, you are absorbing the beneficial energetic properties of that particular substance and not its biochemistry. Many mainstream scientists have argued in favour of energy medicine at great cost to their reputations within the orthodox community, nervous of its implications and therefore doubly sceptical of the evidence supporting it.

One example of scientific persecution is that of scientist Jacques Benveniste, whose research into the memory of water provided an explanation for how homeopathy works. He demonstrated that the molecular organization of water can both store and play back the chemical information of any molecules it once contained. One of his experiments showed that if solutions of antibodies are diluted repeatedly until they are no longer chemically or biologically detectable, the solution still produces a response from the immune cells. This directly contradicts current laws of biochemistry. Benveniste was ridiculed and his research institute closed down — it appears that witch hunts are not confined to history. While such prejudice persists, complementary practitioners will be denied the opportunity to prove that natural healing works not just on a biochemical level but also on a bioelectromagnetic one.

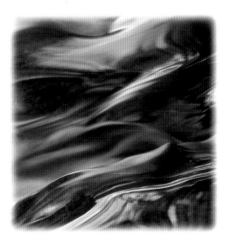

Nature's Beauty Store

The following examples show how you can beautify yourself using Nature's bounty. Wherever possible look for sources that are organic and as unadulterated as possible.

Gentle, regular exfoliation of the dead top layers of skin not only helps slough off that dry, powdery look but stimulates production of fresh, new skin cells and that ensures body products are absorbed more effectively. Pumice stones are excellent for removing the hard skin from the feet. A loofah can be used over the whole body. When applied in upward strokes to the upper thighs, a loofah stimulates the blood and lymphatic circulation to help reduce or eliminate cellulite.

To refine and smooth the skin you can use the soft flesh of a ripe papaya, which contains an enzyme that dissolves the hardened protein, or keratin, that makes skin look rough. Simply cut off a large chunk of papaya, remove the seeds and rub the fleshy part over your clean face and neck. Leave for two minutes, then rinse off with warm water and pat dry.

If you have ever compared the experience of using a natural sponge (the fibrous skeleton of an aquatic creature) with that of the manufactured variety, you will undoubtedly have found the former to be superior, but without knowing why. For most people there is an indefinable quality about using items from Earth's store cupboard for health and beauty. Human beings have been doing so ever since Palaeolithic tribespeople used natural earth pigments to ceremonially paint their bodies.

Before looking at how you can utilize some of these things to enhance your wellbeing, let's examine scientifically why they are so beneficial. The tool which researchers have used is called corona discharge, or Kirlian photography. This process uses high frequencies and streams of electrons to produce pictures of the usually invisible electromagnetic radiation, or auras, of people as well as foods and seeds. Such photographs, where "vitality" resembles iron filings around a magnet, have

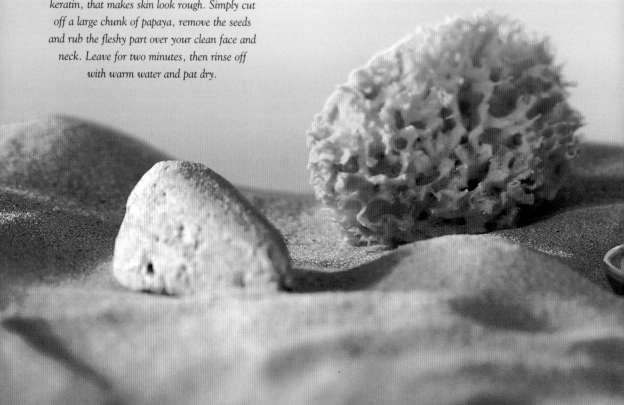

been used to demonstrate, for example, the implications on health of eating highly processed or cooked foods compared with their organic or raw equivalent. Kirlian pioneer and medical researcher, Harry Oldfield, has produced a catalogue of illustrations showing the dramatic difference between the almost non-existent Kirlian field of a subject on a junk food diet compared with a wholefood diet; between the vibrancy of corona discharge of virgin olive oil and that of refined lard.

Similarly, the energy fields of sponges, loofahs, pumice stones, pure essential oils, clay, mud and salts reveal their extension of the electromagnetic field and environmental influence of the Earth from which they came. Because of this, the quality of an object's corona is picked up by the innate sensitivity of the frequencies within and around our physical bodies. This either has a positive or a negative effect on it, a phenomenon also illustrated by Kirlian photography.

Stimulate the body's natural waste disposal system to eliminate toxins built up from our over-processed diet and polluted lifestyle by taking a regular Epsom salts bath (though not if you have high blood pressure). Add two handfuls of these earth minerals to a warm bath and soak for at least 30 minutes. The magnesium and sulphate molecules in the salts help leach out waste materials from the body, at the same time neutralizing and balancing your electrical field.

Plant oils are one of the best ways of gently removing the impurities and grime of modern urban life. Because of their efficient but gentle action they help to get rid of dead skin cells and toxins that can clog pores and cause blemishes, while leaving the skin feeling naturally soft and supple. Try massaging sweet almond or jojoba oil all over your face. Soak a piece of muslin or towelling in hot water (as high a temperature as you can stand), wring it out and thoroughly wipe away all remains of dirt and make-up. You will need to rinse out the cloth and repeat this several times.

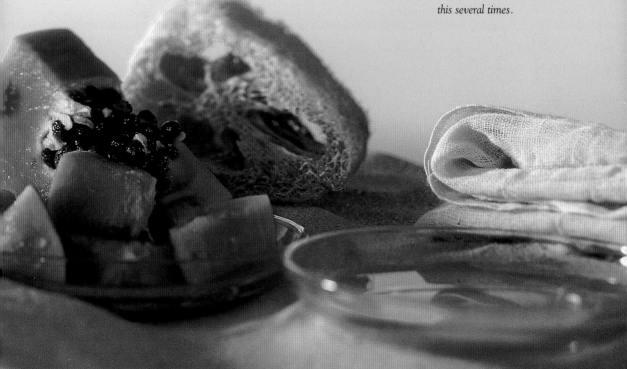

Cleansing and Moisturizing

Honey is a great cleanser and helps to remove dead skin cells that contribute to flaky, lack-lustre skin. Simply massage in, remove with a hot, wrung-out face cloth, and repeat the rinsing process until all dirt and honey are removed.

Bathtime can become an enhanced cleansing and relaxing experience by adding dried herbs or flowers (chamomile or lavender) to warm water, vinegar (great for easing aching muscles), or two handfuls of non-fat milk powder (to help soothe and calm rough or sore skin). Try essential oil blends to help you enjoy a variety of emotional and psychological benefits, particularly through inhaling the active constituents, as you soak.

One of the best ways of cleansing your entire system — enhancing the look and feel of your skin in the process — is to drink 6-8 glasses of pure mineral water every day.

The natural ageing process, with its hormonal shifts, combined with environmental pollutants and the harsh chemicals in everyday household products, including soaps, conspire to rob our skins of vital moisture. We constantly lose moisture in the form of water and natural oils, both in humid conditions and centrally heated environments. Unfortunately air conditioning can undermine hydration levels. To protect and enhance the hydro-lipidic film of our bodies we need to moisturize it regularly.

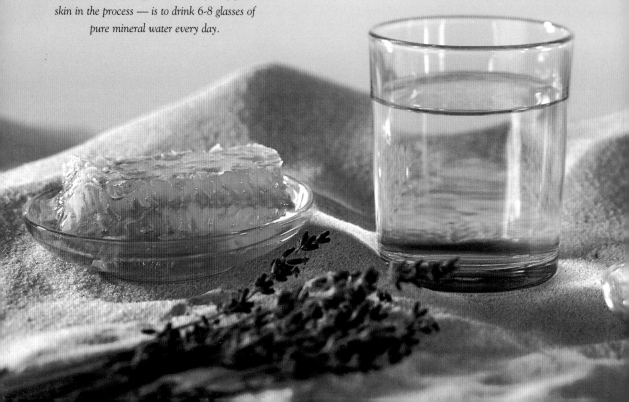

There is a plethora of manufactured products that can help, from petroleum jelly to the most advanced, expensive skin serums. However, your store cupboard contains some beneficial skin treatments, too, which are particularly suitable for those with sensitive skin who have problems with the fragrances and other sensitizers added to shop-bought products.

Mashed avocado — with flesh that contains almost 50 per cent natural oils — can be applied to a dehydrated face to give it a moisture boost. Once you have cleansed and exfoliated your skin, apply the avocado as a mask and leave on for 10-15 minutes, then rinse off thoroughly with warm water.

Oatmeal in the form of porridge oat flakes, from any supermarket, is renowned as a moisturizer for dry, irritated, or sensitive skin. Added to a warm bath it will offer a soothing, if rather messy, experience.

If your hair has becoming dehydrated due to over-use of perming lotions, colorants, the effect of strong sunshine, hairdryers and styling appliances, give it a moisturization boost by massaging in a small quantity of olive or coconut oil. Put on a plastic hair cap after application and leave the oil on the hair for as long as possible, preferably overnight. Bear in mind that you will need several washes, using a mild, frequent-use shampoo, to remove all the oil residue.

Plant oils are some of the most useful moisturizers around. Rub sweet almond oil into clean skin before soaking in a warm relaxing bath. After patting dry there will be no need to add any more creams. Similarly, add a few drops of wheatgerm or carrot oil to your everyday moisturizer to give your skin added suppleness and softness.

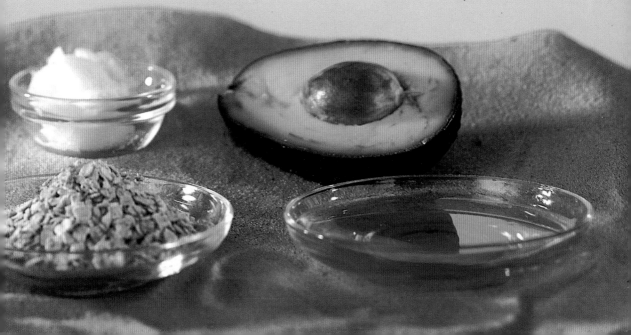

Crystal Healing

Beliefs about the mystical and healing powers of minerals and precious stones, the Earth's bounty, date back to the dawn of history, and are embraced by all cultures. (The chart on pages 148-9 brings together all aspects of using crystals for body layouts, aesthetic pleasure, and meditation/visualization exercises.)

Crystal healing works on the principle that every cell in the body vibrates at its own specific frequency. When these natural frequencies become unbalanced we experience disease. This concept, understood thousands of years ago by intuitive healers within the field of Ayurvedic medicine, for example, is becoming more and more accepted within orthodox medical traditions.

Crystals, in keeping with all else in the Universe, vibrate. When powered by an external source such as a small battery or the Sun, micro-thin slices of synthetic quartz crystals emit very precise electronic pulses, which are then channelled through microchip circuitry to keep time accurately in quartz watches. Thought is also energetic. It is believed that through the power of strong

"Nature has never made two human beings, two plants or two crystals exactly alike. Consider the magnitude of that diversity."
Barbara Walker, The Book of Sacred Stones

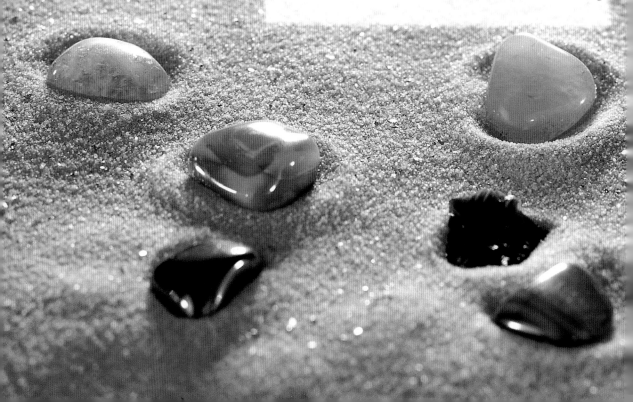

intention — either that of yourself or a crystal therapist — healing energy from an inexplicable force (commonly called the Universal Life Force) is channelled through the crystal to stimulate, balance, or tranquillize your life energy, or chi. In this way crystals can help harmonize and balance the body's natural frequencies back to optimum, healthy levels.

Crystals can be used on many levels. They act as a catalyst for self-healing on the physical, emotional, mental, and spiritual levels and assist the understanding that we each have a very important and profound part to play in our wellbeing. Not everyone resonates with crystals — if nothing else these flowers of the mineral kingdom are powerful symbols of the beauty, mystery, and uniqueness of Earth's bounty.

Grounding crystals

With the contemporary emphasis on intellectualization, many of us experience life "in our heads". Yet spiritual masters stress the importance of maintaining some form of "grounding" or "earthing", in order to fully participate as a human being. Many crystals, particularly those resonating with the red/brown colour associated with the root chakra, can help you to become more rooted in the here and now. Try keeping a small tumblestone in your purse or pocket, or wear a piece of jewellery incorporating any of the following crystals:

Agate, Hematite, Rose quartz, Bloodstone, Carnelian, Smoky quartz, Tiger's eye, Rhodochrosite, Obsidian

Crystal Healing Chart

CHAKRA WORK

CHAKRA	1st Root	2nd Sacral	3rd Solar plexus	4th Heart	5th Throat	6th Third eye	7th Crown
COLOUR	Red, brown, or black	Orange	Yellow	Green, pink	Blue	Indigo	White/Gold
CRYSTALS	Bloodstone, Hematite, Tiger's eye	Citrine, Carnelian, Golden topaz	Sunstone, Smoky quartz, Citrine	Rose quartz, Aventurine quartz, Watermelon tourmaline	Lapis lazuli, Turquoise, Aquamarine	Sodalite, Amethyst, Fluorite	Clear quartz, Diamond, Amethyst

TUNING/DEDICATING

Switching on to a specific purpose

Healing	Meditation	Dream interpretation

Cleansing

Water	Sunlight	Moonlight	Smudging	Earth burial	Amethyst bed	Thought visualization

CHOOSING

Colour	Intuition		Shape			Size: Tumblestones	Size: Larger pieces		
	"Resonance"					Body layouts		Energy clearing, Whole rooms	Sacred space
Links with chakras			Single terminators	Double terminators	Clusters		Meditative focus		
	Mental affinity	Physical tingling							

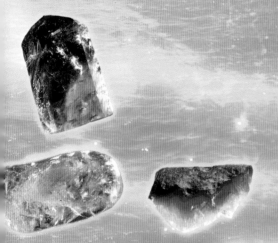

CRYSTAL HEALING

GENERAL PURPOSE

Healing	Aesthetic pleasure	Meditation/visualization
	Releases natural "feel good" brain chemicals	
		Focus
Physical Mental Emotional Spiritual		

Sacred Space

You might like to draw together some of the concepts introduced in this book, to enable you to create your own sacred space. This will be a regular retreat where you can focus on your connection with Earth. It does not need to be grand or complicated; in fact, the smaller and simpler it is, the more likely you will feel that this is your special place, with the advantage that it will not take much time or energy to maintain. A window box or a small corner of your backyard will be perfect.

The step-by-step guide to establishing your sacred space (see right) is intended for inspiration only. As with any journey, the specific route you take is determined by your personal needs. You may choose to decorate your space with beautiful crystals or seasonal flowers, with a statue or a favourite plant or bush. One of the important things to remember is that we empower ourselves every time we take the time to listen to our intuition. In doing so we take responsibility for our lives, even in small ways, until we eventually trust that what we want for ourselves — not what others want for us — is the path to true enlightenment. Therefore, be inspired to place in your sacred space things that are meaningful to you, and to you alone.

1. Meditate on what your sacred space might look like. Play around with the design — what would you like to grow or keep there?

2. Start collecting things that are important to you, or attract you — they must be weather-proof to withstand Sun, rain, frost, and high winds. You could explore a particular theme that reflects spiritual beliefs, do colour work on your chakras, or simply create a collection of favourite plants. Be guided by your intuition.

3. Follow the instructions on dowsing (see pp.86-7), in order to identify the most energizing spot for your sacred space.

4. Once you have found your desired location, acknowledge the Earth devas (see pp.130-1) and ask for their help in clearing away any debris, weeds, or extraneous plants. If possible, wait a season to see what else is growing before finalizing plans. Try to take an "all seasons" perspective, so that your space looks beautiful all year.

5. Avoid overcrowding your space and allow for new items you are drawn to — a crystal, for example, or a water feature. As you change and grow, so too will your sacred space. Decide on regular times to devote to your sacred space and meditate on your relationship with Earth.

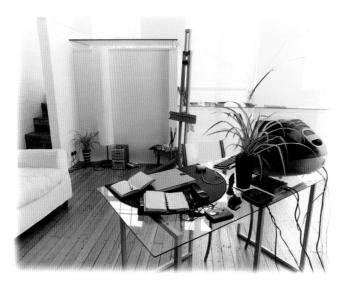

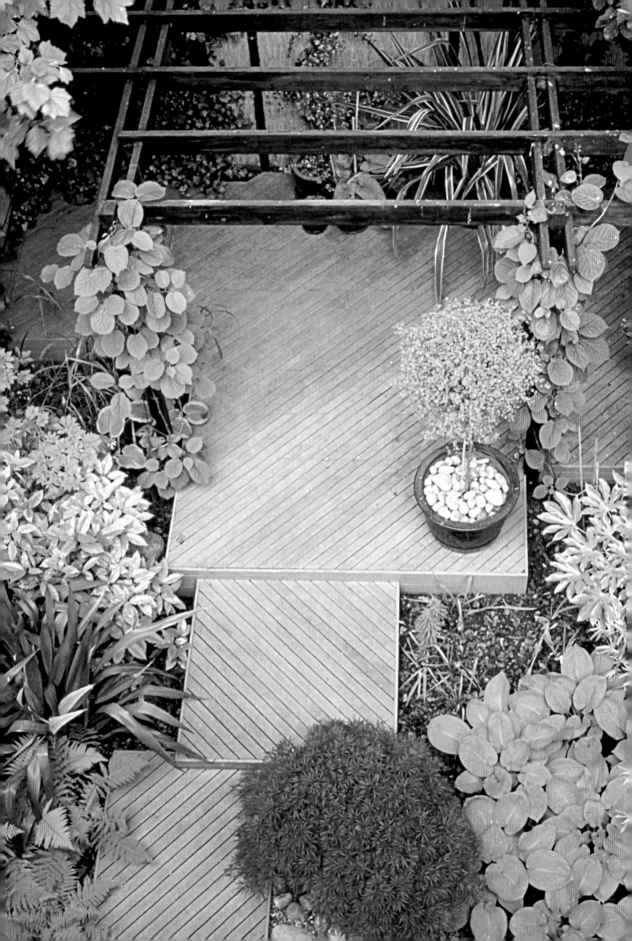

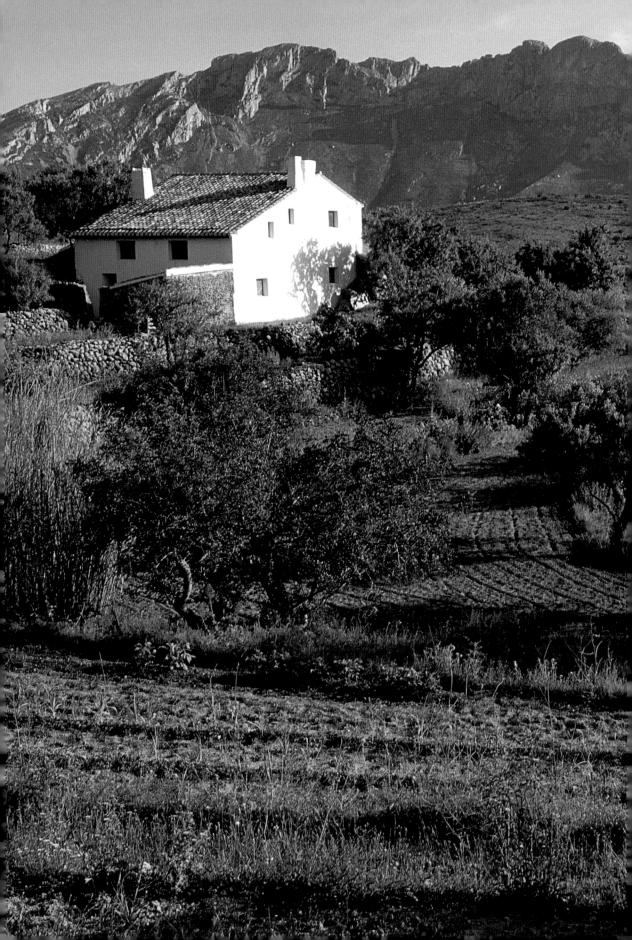

Afterword

One of my favourite affirmations is the one stating that every day we have something to teach and something to learn. Writing this book has been a cathartic experience, helping me to reconnect with my inner self as well as my environment. As such I have developed a greater appreciation for the home in which I live, the garden which provides me with so much joy throughout the seasons, and the important contribution I can make to the future of this planet. I do this by actively choosing to boycott genetically modified and irradiated foods, taking an organic approach to gardening, and generally respecting Gaia, Mother Earth.

As I complete this book, I read that, throughout Europe, depression accounts for almost one-quarter of all illnesses and is currently more widespread than infectious diseases and malnutrition. In the developing world the situation is thought to be even more acute, although exact figures do not exist. I believe the reason behind the alarming wave of depression and general malaise lies with our disassociation from the energy of this planet. I hope that in some small way I have inspired and motivated you to choose to reconnect with Gaia and in so doing that you enjoy greater physical, psychological, and spiritual health and wellbeing.

Love and light,

Liz Simpson, Summer 1999

Resources

Bach flower remedies
Nelson Bach USA, Ltd.
Wilmington Technology Park
100 Research Drive
Wilmington, MA 01887-4406
(800) 334-0843

Flower Essence Society
PO Box 1769
Nevada City, CA 95959
(916) 265-0258
mail@flowersociety.org
www.flowersociety.org

Crystal healing
The Crystal Academy of
Advanced Healing Arts
PO Box 1334
Kapaa, HI 96746
(808) 823-6959

Dowsing
American Society of
Dowsers
PO Box 24
Danville, VT 05828
(800) 711-9530

Feng shui
Feng Shui Warehouse
PO Box 3005
San Diego, CA 92163

Feng Shui Institute of America
PO Box 488
Wabasso, FL 32970

Gardening
Permaculture Institute of
North America
6488 Maxwelton Road
Clinton, WA 98236

Regenerative Agriculture
Association
222 Main Street
Emmaus, PA 18049

The Resources of International
Permaculture
7781 Lenox Avenue
Jacksonville, FL 32221

Meditation
Insight Meditation Society
1230 Pleasant Street
Barre, MA 01005
(617) 355-4378

Spirit Rock
5000 Sir Francis Drake
Boulevard
PO Box 909
Woodacre, CA 94973
(415) 488-0164

Zen Center of San Francisco
300 Page Street
San Francisco, CA 94102
(415) 863-3136

Shamanic healing
Dancing Bear Alternative
Health Center
1000 Fremont Avenue
Suite 150C
Los Altos, CA 95134
(650) 947-8980
www.dancing-bear.com

Spiritual healing
Spiritual Healing Common
Boundary, Inc.
7005 Florida Street
Chevy Chase, MD 20815

Order of the Ascending Spirit
9120 Gramercy Drive #317
San Diego, CA 92123-4010
(615) 560-9228
www.dharma-haven.org/oas

Bibliography

Andrews, Ted, *Animal Speak: The spiritual and magical powers of creatures great and small,* Llewellyn Publications, 1993

Ban Breathnach, Sarah, *Simple Abundance: A daybook of comfort and joy,* Warner Books, 1995

Becklake, Sue, *The Official London Planetarium Book of Space,* Virgin Books, 1994

Bender, Lionel, *Our Planet: A guide to our world and its changing environment,* Simon and Schuster, 1991

Berthon, Simon & Robinson, Andrew, *The Shape of the World: The mapping & discovery of the Earth,* George Philip Ltd, 1991

Bolen, Jean Shinoda, *Goddesses in Everywoman: A new psychology of women,* HarperCollins, 1985

Brunsden, D., *et al, Landshapes,* David & Charles, 1988

Bunyard, P. (ed.), *Gaia in Action,* Floris Books, 1997

Buzan, Tony, *Use Your Memory,* BBC Books, 1986

Buzan, Tony & Keene, Raymond, *Buzan's Book of Genius,* Stanley Paul, 1994

Capra, Fritjof, *The Web of Life,* Doubleday, 1997

Capra, Fritjof, *The Turning Point,* Bantam Doubleday Dell, 1988

Chopra, Deepak, *The Seven Spiritual Laws of Success,* Amber-Allen Publishing and New World Library, 1995

Crowley, Vivianne, *Principles of Paganism,* Thorsons, 1996

Crowley, Vivianne, *Principles of Wicca*, Thorsons, 1998

Curott, Phyllis W., *Book of Shadows*, Broadway, 1998

Dorling Kindersley Science Encyclopaedia, The, DK, 1998

Eiby, G. A., *Earthquakes*, Heinemann Educational Books, 1980

Evans, Ivor H., *Brewer's Dictionary of Phrase & Fable*, HarperCollins, 1995

Farndon, John, *How the Earth Works*, Reader's Digest, 1992

Foods That Harm, Foods That Heal, Reader's Digest, 1996

Gregory, Richard L. (ed.), *The Oxford Companion to the Mind*, Oxford University Press, 1987

Guinness Book of Answers, The, 10th edition, Guinness Publishing Ltd., 1995

Guinness Book of Records 1999, The, Guinness Publishing Ltd, 1999

Harner, Michael, *The Way of the Shaman*, HarperSanFrancisco, 1990

Ions, Veronica, *The History of Mythology*, AAA, 1999

Kenton, Leslie, *The New Joy of Beauty*, Vermilion, 1995

Kingfisher Visual Factfinder, The, Kingfisher Books, 1993

Land, George & Jarman, Beth, *Breakpoint and Beyond: Mastering the future today*, Leadership 2000 Inc.

Lawlor, Robert, *Sacred Geometry: Philosophy and practice*, Thames & Hudson, 1989

Linn, Denise, *Sacred Space: Clearing and enhancing the energy of your home*, Ballantine Books, 1996

Litvinoff, Miles, *The Young Gaia Atlas of Earthcare*, Checkmark Books, 1996

Lovelock, James, *Gaia: The practical science of planetary medicine*, Trans-Atlantic Publications, 1991

Michell, John, *The Earth Spirit: Its ways, shrines and mysteries*, Thames & Hudson, 1975

Michell, John, *The New View Over Atlantis*, Thames & Hudson, 1995

Mitton, Simon & Jacqueline, *The Young Oxford Book of Astronomy*, Oxford University Press, 1998

Molyneaux, Brian Leigh, *The Sacred Earth*, Macmillan Reference Books, 1995

Moore, Alanna, *Divining Earth Spirit*, Alanna Moore, 1994

Orr, Emma Restall, *Principles of Druidry*, Thorsons, 1999

Philip, Neil, *The Illustrated Book of Myths, Tales and Legends of the World*, DK, 1995

Reader's Digest, *How Was it Done?*, Reader's Digest, 1998

Reader's Digest, *Folklore, Myths and Legends of Britain*, Reader's Digest, 1977

Roney-Dougal, Serena, *Where Science and Magic Meet*, Element Books, 1993

Rutherford, Leo, *Principles of Shamanism*, Thorsons, 1997

Saunders, Nicholas J., *Animals' Spirits* (Living Wisdom Series), Time Life Books/Duncan Baird Publishers, 1995

Schiff, Michel, *The Memory of Water*, Thorsons, 1998

Simpson, Liz, *The Book of Crystal Healing*, Sterling Publications, 1997

Simpson, Liz, *The Book of Chakra Healing*, Sterling Publications, 1999

Simpson, Liz, *Working from the Heart: How to love what you do for a living*, Vermilion, 1999

St James, Elaine, *Living the Simple Life: A guide to scaling down and enjoying more*, Hyperion, 1998

Swan, James, *The Power of Place & Human Environments* (anthology), Theosophical Publishing House, 1991

Vitebsky, Piers, *The Shaman*, Little Brown, 1995

Whitfield, P. (ed.), *Our Mysterious Planet: Mysteries of the natural world*, Cassell, 1990

Wildwood, Chrissie, *The Encyclopedia of Healing Plants: A guide to aromatherapy, flower essences and herbal remedies*, Piatkus, 1998

Index

*Main entries are in **bold**.*

Photography

Bernard Boullet 2, 6, 8, 9, 12-13, 14, 15, 45, 46, 55, 59, 60, 80, 81, 83, 85, 88, 98-9, 100, 101, 107, 113, 114-15, 124, 132, 133, 139, 140, 152
David Cavagnaro 24, 27, 28-9, 30, 34-5, 39, 65, 93, 102-3, 104-5, 110-11
Adrian Swift 142-3, 144-5, 146-7
Dominic Blackmore 116-17, 118-19, 120-1, 122-3, 150
Photodisc 18, 19, 20, 21, 22-3, 26, 31, 32, 33, 38, 42, 44, 50-1, 70, 79, 141
Werner Forman Archive 61, 62-3, 67, 68-9, 71, 75, 76-7
The Garden Picture Library 86-7, 126-7, 128-9, 151

Julie Williams (illustrations) 86-7, 118-19, 120-1, 126

Acknowledgements

Author's acknowledgements
This book represents the accumulation of knowledge as well as the support and motivation I have received from many special people. They know who they are. For this I offer my heartfelt thanks and love. But I'd like to particularly mention my editor at Gaia, Jo Godfrey Wood and the design team of Matt Moate and Sara Mathews. Here's to the further success of a winning team!

Publisher's acknowledgements
Gaia Books would like to thank the following individuals for their help in producing this book: Lynn Bresler (proofreading and indexing), Cathy Meeus (proofreading), and Patrick Nugent.

If you liked *The Healing Energies of Earth*, you should read:

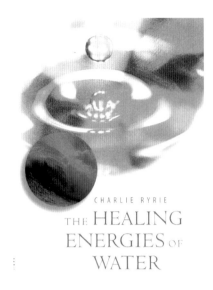

THE HEALING ENERGIES OF WATER
by Charlie Ryrie

This book explores the human relationship with water throughout
the centuries, explains water's importance for the health of the
body, outlines different water remedies for a variety of ailments,
and, finally, suggests how to use energized water in the home
or garden for health, meditation, and relaxation.

ISBN 1-885203-72-1

CHARLIE RYRIE

THE HEALING
ENERGIES OF
WATER

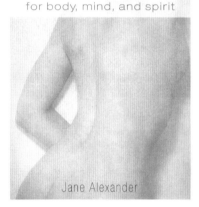

THE DETOX PLAN
FOR BODY, MIND, AND SPIRIT
by Jane Alexander

The Detox Plan is a clear, simple, and definitive
guide to ridding yourself of unwanted toxins,
clutter, and negative thoughts. It offers readers
easy, practical ways to integrate healthy living
into even the most hectic lifestyles.

ISBN 1-885203-70-5

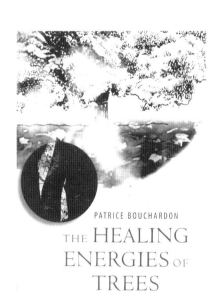

THE HEALING ENERGIES OF TREES
by Patrice Bouchardon

The Healing Energies of Trees offers readers the potential to harness
the power of trees for self-healing and personal development and
transformation. Readers discover how to connect with trees, and
how this intimacy can help resolve their physical and emotional
problems, and become a catalyst for their creativity.

ISBN 1-885203-71-3

PATRICE BOUCHARDON

THE HEALING
ENERGIES OF
TREES

For a complete catalog, call or write:
Tuttle Publishing/Journey Editions, Airport Industrial Park, 364 Innovation Drive, North Clarendon, VT 05759-9436
phone: (802) 773-8930 • fax: (802) 773-6993 • toll-free: (800) 526-2778